Enabling future care

Michele Moore and Judd Skelton with Martin Patient

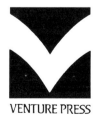

VENTURE PRESS

BASW website: http://www.basw.co.uk

Published by
VENTURE PRESS
16 Kent Street
Birmingham
B5 6RD

British Library Cataloguing-in-Publication Data
A catalogue record for this book is available from the British Library

ISBN 1–86178–039–7 (paperback)

Design, layout and production by
Hucksters Advertising & Publishing Consultants,
Riseden, Tidebrook,
Wadhurst, East Sussex TN5 6PA

Cover design by
Western Arts, 194 Goswell Road
London, EC1V 7DT

Printed and bound in Great Britain by Biddles Ltd,
www.biddles.co.uk

Contents

Acknowledgements

The original ideas for this book arose through the shared experiences of people with learning difficulties and older caregivers connected with Sale and Altrincham MENCAP and their chosen ally Martin Patient, a voluntary sector worker with long experience of trying to support families grappling with older care issues.

Martin's commitment to pioneering advocacy of rights and opportunities for disabled people and their families enabled funding to be obtained from Salford and Trafford Health Authority to access the aspirations of older caregivers and people with learning difficulties with whom they live. Many people contributed to the ensuing project which is the main focus of this book and, while it is not possible to mention everyone by name, we have benefited from their support and encouragement. Most of all, we would like to thank the families who so generously assisted with our enquiries. They will know who they are and we thank them for the characteristic warmth with which the researchers were welcomed into their lives. We are indebted to fellow researchers, Sarah Beazley and June Maelzer who were members of the original project team. The ongoing work and publications of Carol Walker at Sheffield Hallam University, John Harris of the British Institute of Learning Disabilities and Dan Goodley of the University of Leeds have been significant in our thinking.

Notes about the text

PEOPLE WITH LEARNING DIFFICULTIES

We use the specific term people with learning difficulties in order to take seriously opinions and preferences which have been articulated through the self-advocacy movement:

> *If you put 'people with learning difficulties', then they know that people want to learn and to be taught how to do things.*
>
> **(self advocate, quoted in Sutcliffe and Simons, 1993 p.23)**

CAREGIVERS

We use the term caregiver because, as pointed out by Morris (1993), the definition of a person as a 'carer' is impossible to sustain in everyday life. There is reciprocity of support, love and help within family life. The term caregiver helps to affirm this. To clarify:

> *In the context of the political professional and academic debates on community care, 'care' – whether it refers to people giving paid or unpaid help – does not mean to 'care about' someone in the sense of loving them. Rather it means to 'care for' someone in the sense of taking responsibility for them.*
>
> **(Morris, 1993 p.149)**

SOURCES

Unless otherwise stated, all quotations and inserts are caregivers or practitioners talking to members of our Disability Research Team (Skelton et al., 1997). The source of an inclusion is indicated if it has come from elsewhere or, on a few occasions, if specific clarification is warranted.

Introduction

> *Parents and people who choose to care for someone are the most dedicated people I have met. What better service provision could there be? These people should be given the respect, support and finances that they need.*
>
> **Social worker**

WHAT THIS BOOK IS ABOUT

In this book we aim to encourage service providers to reflect on their work with older caregivers and people with learning difficulties. Its recommendations will be invaluable to anyone involved in community care services, including service users.

Our enquiries, and analysis of other research, have uncovered many stories of struggle which depict caregivers and people with learning difficulties as faced with continual and uphill battles to create change which is rooted in their immediate and practical concerns. Yet those who contributed to this book are not content to blame policy or individual practitioners and do not paint an entirely gloomy picture of their situations. They make suggestions for practitioners and policy-makers which reflect their experiences of positive intervention and support. They understand the role policy plays in shaping practice. Their concern is to move their struggle beyond their own resources and capacities by inviting practitioners to work collaboratively with them. They seek to make *their* perspective create the knowledge and practices which shape their experiences and we have treated this as the primary aim of this book.

That this previously neglected area of family support is under consideration at all shows there is currently real potential for change. A good indication of the

Government's increasing recognition of the entitlements of caregivers can be found in the National Carers Strategy (1999) published by the Department of Health.

What carers do should be properly recognised, and properly supported – and the Government should play its part. Carers should be able to take pride in what they do. And in turn, we should take pride in carers. I am determined to see that they do – and that we all do.
Prime Minister, Rt. Hon. Tony Blair, 1999

The rights and entitlements of people with learning difficulties are also gaining increased respect largely through the efforts of the rapidly expanding self-advocacy movement which has begun to forge widespread recognition of the resilience of people with learning difficulties (Goodley, 1997; 1998; Skelton and Moore, 1999).

The theme of 'resilience' is an important one throughout this book. Much of the material is steeped in practical concerns about how best caregivers and the people they support can challenge assumptions made by practitioners, or circumvent service philosophies and practices which regulate their experiences in negative ways. But the book is more than a user-led protest about service provision. What makes it meaningful as a guide for practitioners is the value which service users place on providers who they perceive to be 'getting it right'. The stories which are at the heart of our analysis help to make plain what 'getting it right' consists of in the eyes of ageing caregivers and people with learning difficulties.

We are just beginning to learn about how families combine family life with care commitments (Kagan and Lewis, 1996; Lewis et al, 1999), but relatively little research relates to older caregivers and people with learning difficulties. What this neglect may mean is that these groups are on the receiving end of policy decisions which are arbitrary in terms of underlying assumptions. Service delivery comes across as indifferent if their right to have a meaningful say gets overlooked.

Many older caregivers have told us that while they want to talk about, and need to plan for the future, they are providing care *now* and they need support *now*. Because they are getting older, they may need more support than previously. This does not mean that they cannot cope or want to plan for the future straightaway: just that they need practitioners to think about ways which will help them to carry on. Effective input for people in their current circumstances enriches future care possibilities. Sometimes it is easy to be hasty and think *'right, they're struggling, it's time for the move,'* when in fact with a little extra support, they can continue if that is what all the family wants. Helping families to plan for the future is important but so is supporting them in their current caregiving arrangements. Others are clear that they do not want to be maintained in their caregiver role and that their sons and daughters do not want to remain dependent on them but want individual and independent lives.

The least we can do to reassert their rights is to listen to what they say.

Agendas and aspirations

LISTENING TO CAREGIVERS

We found this talk given by an older caregiver, transformed our thinking[1]:

I would like to introduce myself. I'm Vic Riley, I come from Wigan, that's me, and I'm married to Sylvia. I met Sylvia probably thirty-four, thirty-five years ago and we will have been married thirty years in October. In that period of time we've had 3 sons, Stuart, Timothy and Robert. Stuart's my oldest son. He's really into fast cars and really into fast women, I think. Tim, my middle son, is into motorbikes and he's settled down with his partner Sarah, and Robert likes motorbikes as well, and he's not yet bothered about women, he likes the manly things. All my sons are men. Stuart's twenty-seven, Tim's twenty-six and Robert's twenty-five. Stuart and Robert, my first and third son, are also known as people who have a severe learning disability and Robert, my youngest son, has just about every label it's possible to have. I guess any mums and dads who have disabled sons or daughters, soon after their child was born, have thought 'who's going to look after my sons and daughters when anything happens to me?'. What I decided I would talk about is around partnership and around planning.

Tim and Stuart and Robert all moved out of our house at about the same time. Tim moved out with his partner, Sarah, and bought a new house. Stuart and Robert moved into a house that we picked, Stuart, Robert, Sylvia and myself, with Tim and Sarah. We chose it just a few minutes away from Sylvia and my house, about four minutes walk. It's just an ordinary house. It isn't specially adapted in any way. It's a house which a small builder built and we got a Housing Association to buy it. Stuart and Robert moved in as tenants in that house, so that they have all the legal rights of living in that house. Stuart and Robert have twenty-four hour support and that is by a staff team or a team of enablers, who are employed by an organisation called The Wigan Link.

The Wigan Link, when it started, was a group of mums and dads who had sons or daughters who happened to have a learning disability. The Wigan Link started because a group of us came together and decided we didn't want to accept the future that we had seen other families experience. We wanted more opportunities and more options than they had. We wanted to plan, so that ➤

◀ when the time was right for our sons and our daughters they could move out of the family home and set up in their own homes.

The Wigan Link is an on-going group. We've just got some funding through the lottery and taken on a development worker who is doing some lifestyle planning with quite a number of people. We're a charity, we're not looking to make any profits. We're looking for any money that comes into The Wigan Link to go to the individuals we're supporting. It's a company limited by a guarantee – that is simply a safeguard in case anything did go wrong and money had gone missing. We're all responsible for a share and that's all and it's made up of family members, because although I said we started with mums and dads, we now have brothers and sisters involved with the management group. We're looking very much to support the principles of an ordinary life, with ordinary opportunities.

I would like one thing to be on my grave stone when I'm dead. I would like it to be that I had a dream for my sons. For each and every one of my sons, not just for Tim, my middle son. When Stuart and Robert lived at home with us, each of them had a certain dream, and we used to talk a lot about things and how it can be, and my dream, for the future for Stuart and for Robert was that they continue to have a good life. That their life is as ordinary as can be, because there is a lot of value in an ordinary life. My dream was for Stuart and Robert, when the time was right, to move into their own home, that they have been included in choosing, and live with people who they would want to live with and who want to live with them. My dream is that the values that they are surrounded by are ordinary family values. Respect is vitally important, so that Stuart and Robert are seen as people first, so they are included in any decisions that are made, as if when they still lived with us.

I hope to be included in my son's lives as long as I am alive, but not always as a member of the group The Wigan Link. I'm the Chair of The Wigan Link but it's essential that we learn the lesson of bringing younger people in to take over for when we can no longer do it. Younger family members who will work to keep The Wigan Link going are important and will ensure that the people with learning difficulties who are being supported will have the best and that family values will run on. It pays to take turns doing the hard jobs, and the question of who we can trust is important. Because traditionally, and although I'm talking about partnerships and it is essential to build partnerships with the local authority, with the health authority, with other voluntary organisations, it is difficult to know who you can trust. I trust my family, and I trust other people who have had the same sorts of problems through their life as I've had. So I trust parents first, not professionals; the history of our group has taught me that. The message I am trying to get across is that really I think everybody needs to pull together. When you see geese heading South for the winter, flying along in a V-formation, it is interesting to think about why they fly that way. Scientists have discovered that as each bird flaps its wings it creates an uplift for the bird ▶

≪ immediately following it. Flying in a V-formation the whole flock has at least seventy-one per cent flying uplift. And there is a lesson to be learned from that. The lesson is that people who share a common direction and have a sense of common direction can get where they're going quicker and easier by travelling on the strengths of each other. If we've got the sense of geese, then service providers, policy makers and families will all work together like that, to enable and encourage older caregivers and people with learning difficulties in their struggle for control over their future affairs.

Vic Riley's experience raises critical questions about how practitioners can evolve more participatory modes of service planning and delivery. It shows that many families are currently challenging and contesting assumptions about their role in long-term caregiving. They reject narrow and restrictive images of people with learning difficulties as dependent upon their parents for the provision of care. The huge changes in the organisation of family life described provide a powerful indicator of the potential impact of individual and community action in bringing about change. It is not enough just to read this story. It prompts us to make an immediate note of ways in which it challenges images of families involved in caregiving and amplifies our personal understandings of what they face. Some shifts in thinking that we were required to make included:

- trying to get rid of assumptions that families involved in caregiving are somehow 'other' and different from 'ordinary' families;

- recognising that all families are different – there are many variations of family, for example, adoptive families, reconstituted families, separated families, those living with bereavement, having multiple commitments, being determined by particular cultural patterns of extension and so on – we cannot assume sameness simply because the family includes people with learning difficulties and caregivers;

- recognising the limitations of individualising issues and the way in which this intensifies 'problems'.

SOCIAL MODEL OF DISABILITY

Disabled people and their representative organisations say that service providers are at their best when they show through their communications and actions that they understand and accept the *social* nature of disability. As Vic Riley makes clear, it is not helpful for practitioners to think in terms of individual limitations (Barnes, 1990; Morris, 1997; Oliver, 1996; Priestly, 1999). Most people we met made it plain that, in their experience, disability and difficulty are the result of prejudicial actions and discriminatory practices and environments, not individual capacities. Both caregivers and people with learning difficulties can be worn down by services which produce or compound their respective and shared problems. Policy and practice which fail caregivers create uncertainty for people with learning difficulties, and likewise, policy and practice which undermine people with learning difficulties jeopardise the well-being of those who support them.

For example, Kate can speak four languages yet has the sole option of spending her time making party hats in a day centre. Her caregivers know she finds this dispiriting:

> *it's like factory work ... they do it because they have to do it to pass the time ... she can't carry on like this, she needs something stimulating.*

The family knows that if Kate is reluctant to attend the centre then the locus of responsibility will fall on them:

> *something is better than nothing. At least she's got a place there. If they tell us tomorrow there is no place for her we can't do anything.*

The social origins of disablement are plain. In everyday terms, caregivers may not routinely be thought of as 'disabled'. But using the *social model of disability* to interrogate their experience compels us to recognise that caregivers who perceive themselves to be ignored by social services until they can no longer manage, are being incapacitated by prevailing community care practices.

Inadequate service provision for people with learning difficulties, makes caregivers vulnerable too :

> *these carers, every day they are one day older and one of these days there is going to be three of four of them who are going to fold up in an instant because they clearly cannot go on forever ... if you sit in a bath and you increase the temperature by one degree every three hours, when do you jump out saying 'that's scalding': it is probably hot.*

Community care policies and practices for people with learning difficulties and for caregivers have to be viewed as entwined. The entitlements of each group will suggest different priorities for service providers. Each individual must have their personal aspirations and entitlements fully respected. But the fundamentally integrated and enmeshed nature of relations in families where care is an integral dynamic means that planning is not likely to succeed if changes in the interests of one party are made without reference to the interests of the other. This is not an argument for disregarding personal autonomy and individual choice. It is an argument for recognising that personal autonomy and individual choice are, for most people, hardly ever smoothly negotiated without reference to other people's viewpoints.

If, for example, a person with learning difficulties decides they would like to try out Adult Placement, either short term or long term, a number of practitioners will be involved. These include a Care Manager to support the rights and interests of the person with learning difficulties, the prospective new caregivers (perhaps, respite, link or short-term foster carers) and an Adult Placement worker whose role is to support both the interests of those who will be providing shared care and the service user. Other professionals such as physio- or occupational therapists may be involved. However, there is rarely anyone in this process specifically to support, represent and be accountable to the original caregiver(s). While there are many examples of good practice, when practitioners go out of their way to ensure that caregivers are being sufficiently involved and consulted in such a process, caregivers frequently find this is a matter of pot luck and they are relatively powerless. Practitioners faced with this situation will want to encourage links with voluntary sector organisations which can provide representation for caregivers in their own right.

> *The government wants all organisations involved in caring to recognise that they can no longer have a focus just on the client, patient or the user. They must see the person needing care and support within the whole environment of their family, their neighbourhood and their community. This must involve their carer or carers. Statutory services must take an inclusive approach – one which the voluntary sector, in many respects, has been following for a long time.*
>
> **(Blair, 1999)**

It is easy to create difficulty if interventions ignore the social parameters of individual lives. This is why it is important for practitioners to break down the disabling influence of individually focused interventions when working with older caregivers and people with learning difficulties. Successful outcomes for Vic Riley and his family have been achieved through taking an inclusive approach and looking for social, not individual, accountability. The social model of disability implicates a range of conceptual and *practical* changes for practitioners who are serious about maximising support of caregivers and people with learning difficulties (as illustrated in box 1).

Seeking social explanations enables practitioners to set aside theories of individuals as having difficulties which may be hard to get round and makes it possible, instead, to think about ways in which the wider community can be called to account. It then becomes possible to identify the practical actions which need to be taken in order to support people more effectively. Plans for dismantling real barriers can be made out. Working with the social view of disability to remodel support in ways which caregivers and people with learning difficulties prioritise provides the crucial key for

Box 1 Recognizing social dimensions of difficulty

CONCERNS EXPRESSED BY SERVICE USERS	FOCUSING ON INDIVIDUALS LIMITS PRACTITIONERS	FOCUSING ON SOCIAL FACTORS EMPOWERS PRACTITIONERS
'Chris is waking up at three o'clock in the morning and again at half past five in the morning and not going to sleep again during the day because he's just going into the day centre and sitting on a chair all day'	Chris has sleep problems and his caregivers have problems coping with sleep disturbance	What changes can be made in the day centre routine to occupy Chris more adequately? What alternatives can be found to the day centre? How can Chris participate in less sedentary activities – such as sport or performing arts for example?
'I get a report saying David did not want to take part in the beauty session. Well I don't think he does really	David and his caregivers are uncooperative	How can David and his caregivers be more effectively involved in planning?
'We just go our own way now, Tara and me .. you don't really have much happiness in my position because there's not many places where I can really go without Tara'	Tara's mother has low morale and Tara is a millstone around her mother's neck	Are there trusted others or a 'sitting service' who could provide cover while Tara's mother goes out for a while?
'I'm depressed about the new date for Shilpa moving into her Adult Placement. We had agreed the beginning of July and now her Care Manager has changed it to the beginning of May'	Shilpa's caregiver is reluctant to let go whereas Shilpa will feel restricted if her Adult Placement is delayed.	Could someone from a Voluntary organisation represent Shilpa's care giver at planning meetings, alongside Shilpa's Care Manager, to encourage a transition which is more acceptable because it takes into account the feelings of everyone who will be affected by the changes?

achieving excellence in this difficult area of community care. We often hear practitioners say that the social model of disability has been around for a long time now. The evidence of its impact will be realised when every single day-to-day struggle which caregivers and people with learning difficulties face is automatically interrogated by professionals in relation to its social origins.

Some questions worth thinking through

- What do you understand by 'the social origins of disability'?
- From your personal experience, what does it feel like to have the social dimensions of your own problems ignored?
- What are the major implications of this issue for your work?

1. An earlier version of this story appeared in the journal *Community, Work and Family*, 1998. Names have not been changed.

Dreams and reality

It might be assumed that values espoused in major pieces of policy and legislation relating to community care, such as the right to an ordinary life, a home of one's own, personal freedom and choices, can be taken for granted. But many caregivers and people with learning difficulties find these priorities only half-remembered by providing agencies. Aspirations for an ordinary life, a home of one's own, personal freedom and choices are often treated as far-fetched dreams. People tend to draw a line between what they would like and the reality they expect. Yet, mostly, their 'dreams' consist of little more than the preservation of basic human rights and rather ordinary aspirations.

> *That would be a dream, to have a big bungalow, say, with three or four bedrooms ... they must have their own bedroom, they must have their own individuality ... I have it all planned really, and a garden, patio doors leading into a garden where they could sit, with trees for shade or with hammocks.*

Many scenarios we come across, suggest that caregivers frequently have in mind not only the future well-being of their sons or daughters, but also a wider humanitarian agenda concerning the rest of the community. Theirs is an agenda about extending citizenship, enabling ordinary lives and placing value on the family:

> *my future plans for Harry are to leave the house for him to still live in with a possible two other people like himself to share with twenty-four-hour support. We would sell the house to the Housing Association or similar and we would rent property near by. This would be perfect for Harry and the only way I could* ➤

give him up. This house is well adapted for him and would suit anyone who shared with him. A dream maybe, but who knows! I would still be able to visit Harry, sit in the garden with him, maybe take tea with him. I could also have him for weekends and take him on holiday. I would do the respite care instead of social services. I would still have strong contacts with my son.

The arrangements proposed offer benefits not only to one person with learning difficulties but also for two of his peers, their caregivers and family members and for the receiving Housing Association, in respect of adapted property which will bring benefits to the local community in future years. Local authorities have scope for flexibility and discretionary influence over purchasing decisions (Priestly, 1999). Caregivers and people with learning difficulties have specific and viable ideas about how to exploit this and it is beneficial if purchasers are open to their suggestions. Focus on individuals as the recipients of budget allocations imposes dependency and obscures possibilities for developing both citizenship and inclusive communities. Purchasers need to think laterally about outcome measurements:

- do purchasing decisions recognise potential outcomes not only for individual service users, but also quality of life issues for caregivers and value to families and communities?
- if not, what steps have to be taken to ensure that they do?
- what gains will come from widening discussion to include the perspectives of caregivers and people with learning difficulties?

WHAT'S POSSIBLE?

> *Mr W. lives with his son Dan who is in his thirties, and
> who he has supported alone since Dan's mother died.
> Dan has always lived with his family as it was felt
> that there was nowhere else which could provide the
> support he needed.*
>
> *Mr W. has set up a Discretionary Trust, which will
> ensure that while Dan will not directly receive any
> money, trustees will be able to use the money as he
> and Dan would wish. However, as he admits, the
> local authority will have to help out as there is not
> enough money to fund Dan at the amount currently
> projected:* 'Dan is likely to find himself fairly well off,
> but not well enough off, that's the problem.'
>
> *Dan is very well known and very popular in his
> neighbourhood. Mr W. would ideally like Dan to stay
> in his home, after he dies:* 'they could say, well, Dan
> can stay here. We'll bring somebody else in and feed in
> the necessary staffing'.
>
> *However, despite Mr W.'s own attempts at planning, he
> is unable to pin the local authority down to finalising
> arrangements. Even though Mr W. is prepared to hand
> over his house to the local authority, and has set up a
> trust which will be able to finance a substantial
> proportion of Dan's support, he is thwarted by
> inflexibility from the local authority. He feels no
> action will be taken until there is an emergency:* 'I've
> had two heart attacks ... I could drop dead tomorrow,
> and that would simply bring in this activity. There is
> nothing [else] I can do that I haven't done that is
> within my power... I have made every provision, I have
> organised everything that I can. I can't organise it any
> more'.

There is a widespread misconception that families want
'the impossible' and service providers say this makes them
feel relatively helpless. But if the detail of what service
users want is explored and taken seriously, providers can
often find they could deliver more than might at first be
supposed. None of the aspirations uncovered by our

research are really the stuff of dreams but basic requirements. It is worth thinking about what can be done to acknowledge, and thus respect, the aspirations of families more adequately. This, in itself, imposes no millstone around the necks of purchasers.

A sense of being genuinely listened to seems to be the foremost requirement, and the magnitude of what caregivers and people with learning difficulties want in terms of support is not beyond what they might reasonably expect, at least, to talk about.

> *instead of sitting in an office behind a big pile of paper, [practitioners] should get out and meet the family*

Lack of empathy is the most frequent criticism which older caregivers make about practitioners (BILD, 1998).

> *Come and sit and listen to families first. Find out about [my son], spend a bit of time with him, before starting to tell me what I need.*

RESOURCES AND EMPOWERMENT

Caregivers are acutely conscious of resource constraints on support services: *'in every council they all have problems spinning the money out'*. They appreciate that purchasers are hard-pushed to make limited resources stretch and that there are conflicting priorities. But they feel their families are relegated to the bottom of the hierarchy in these struggles. They feel they are viewed *en masse* and that this allows providers to be relatively immune to, and unmoved by, the day-to-day predicaments of families.

> *I mean you take the aged, the aged say that there should be more done for the aged. You talk to the disabled, they feel that more should be done for them. You talk to the out-of-work people, they feel more should be done for them and so it goes on.*

In the eyes of people who have contributed to this book, getting the resources they require comes down to the personal motivation of purchasers and providers to be moved by the urgency of their struggles.

> *Improvements will come from one of two ways. One is for me to win the lottery or secondly for the local authority to realise there is a time bomb waiting... But of course, they don't see our time bomb as really being a problem. They see other time bombs like the education provision or the pavements are collapsing or they need some more roads done or they need some more libraries.*
>
> *I want to feel that they are doing what they should be doing ... because the money **is** there to be paid for these people and they **should** be working to do this job, not to just sit around their office and say 'well, sorry, mate we can't do it' and fob you off.*

Providing caregivers and people with learning difficulties with opportunities to voice their responses to budget decisions and to express their visions for better allocations is of great importance. Many conclude there is wastage of resources because services are not tailored to the families' specific needs and that their role in budget related decision-making is well worth addressing. This requires a willingness of service providers to position themselves as working *with* families and not *for* them, but relinquishing power is still seen by some professionals as difficult:

> *Maybe, you know there should be more control or shared management of teams and social workers and whatever, by parents ... maybe that is a dangerous thing to suggest, that we put carers in charge of the resources.*

Such reservations raise vital questions about how providers respond to – or, conversely, restrict – the role of service users in determining decisions. Families want to have a real say in what support they do get. They do not want promises that cannot be delivered, but they do want delivery of what is promised (Walker and Walker, 1998). Even those who find service providers very helpful and supportive can also recall instances of breakdowns in communication and trust.

- What action can be taken to enable caregivers and people with learning difficulties to contribute to service monitoring and evaluation?
- Are there existing practices which provide for such participation? If not, how can an appropriate strategy be convened? Who could you contact in relation to this? When?

EVOLVING A CLEAR PERSPECTIVE ON BENEFITS AND ENTITLEMENTS

Those parents who are clever, they know how to claim money, but people like me doesn't know anything. If you go and ask them what can you get, they don't tell you, they say 'read this and this pamphlet', and then they tell you another one and they say 'go and get this pamphlet'. When you ring them for the pamphlet you don't find them. So we doesn't know about our rights. We are not that clever that we can ask them for this entitlement or that entitlement.

Questions of what constitutes an adequate income for caregivers, how eligibility for entitlements is perceived and, critically, how much the income of families can be maximised – through state or private means – are hugely complicated. It is helpful if practitioners are mindful of their essential role as individuals who *can* influence understandings of entitlements and assist with challenging barriers to entitlement decisions where this is wanted. Financial insecurity is a major source of stress and distress for people. Finances have to be faced up to and planned for and it ought to be possible for practitioners to ensure easy access to relevant and uncomplicated facts and figures. Professionals, older caregivers and disabled people are unanimous in describing welfare rights as 'a minefield'

and so the main provisions at the time of writing have
been summarised in Appendix I.

> - What promotion materials could be developed for making sure
>   people know about their respective entitlements? What use
>   could be made of formats such as video, audio-tape, parallel
>   text, large print, computer disc and the internet? What expertise
>   exists within your team or department and linked agencies?
>   Who could be invited to join an entitlement promotions team?
>   How would the team benefit from the inclusion of caregivers
>   and people with learning difficulties?
> - In what new ways could information be disseminated about
>   entitlements? What about posters, articles on successful claims
>   in local newspapers, newsletters; short talks on local TV, radio
>   and disability press? Who else could information about
>   entitlements be distributed to? What about caregiver networks
>   and voluntary agencies? What actions can you take to open up
>   some of these avenues for more widely accessible information?
> - What mechanisms can be put in place to ensure that people
>   get *sound* financial advice?
> - How can you keep yourself fully up to date with the latest
>   entitlement issues and provisions? Who can help you?

THE 'HUMAN FACE' OF SERVICE PROVISION

Certain practitioners are repeatedly identified as being the
'human face' of service provision. These people have good
interpersonal skills and an open, warm and empathic manner
which encourages trust. They do not necessarily have a track
record of radically changing service provision or of
extravagant individual commissioning. Often, they are people
who are involved with a family on an ongoing basis but first
impressions are important: *'I know right away whether I like
them or not'*. The most respected practitioners understand
that small things, like phoning when they say they will and
not cancelling meetings, make all the difference.

> *We were sat here, waiting like, and all of a sudden,
> the phone goes. I answered the phone and it was [the
> social worker]. She couldn't come, she'd got
> something more important. I said 'well, as far as I'm
> concerned, there is nothing more important than
> what we want to know'.*

It is significant that the same 'champions of best practice' are nominated by families time and time again. We heard consistently glowing accounts of efforts one particular worker makes to support families in maximising their income. We asked the named person to outline their approach and found they take a great deal of trouble to help make relevant organisations more accessible to disabled people and their allies (Swain *et al*., 1999):

When I am working with a family, I use the basic knowledge I have of welfare rights, but anything slightly complicated, and I am on the phone to Manchester Advice or another appropriate agency. I think probably one of the best things about the welfare rights course I did, wasn't that it gave me a complete working knowledge of every benefit and entitlement, but it did give the understanding of where to go and who I should approach for help on various issues.

I always give people the option of making these calls themselves or me making calls for them. For some caregivers, it can be an empowering experience finding their own way through the information. However, for others, it can be a disempowering one as they come up against different barriers. People vary, and need to be given a choice. There are many caregivers who, I know, would not contact various agencies if it was left to them, as their confidence of finding their way through the system has been so undermined in the past.

I always try to have a contact at any of the places I recommend, so that I am giving those carers who want to do it themselves, a name and also access to someone who I, or other carers, have found to be helpful. I also follow up with calls to caregivers to see how their call went and whether they need any help with anything emerging from the calls, like, help filling in forms. This is also a useful chance to find out about any information that other carers need to know which can be disseminated through our newsletter.

Family Support Worker

The 'best' practitioners:

- work supportively and
- collaboratively,
- challenge constructively,
- handle criticism well and
- engage in more positive communications than their less accepted colleagues.

They position themselves as *a* source of support and make sure they, and the people they work with, are well connected with others. They cannot always make dreams come true, but they have a wide vision of what could potentially become a reality. They put their time and energy into continually opening up new possibilities.

Reconciling dreams and resources

Caregivers and people with learning difficulties express a strong commitment to improving relations with practitioners and so, as part of our research, we organised a one-day workshop to bring them together. The event was evaluated very positively by participants so we have described it is some depth as it may offer a model for similar events elsewhere.

The involvement of people with learning difficulties as informants in evaluations is a relatively new phenomenon and we opted for group discussions as a useful method for accessing their views (Atkinson and Williams, 1990; Booth and Booth, 1994; Rodgers, 1999). Responses were recorded in prose and pictures, in accordance with the wishes expressed by self-advocacy groups, for accessible research processes (for example, *London People First's, 'Making It Easy First' project*, Bashford *et al.*, 1995). The contributions were then typed up, prose and pictures combined, and handed back to respondents for them to check, change, alter, remove or add any information. We took the view that data would only be included in the research analysis when participants said that our account of their perspective was as they wished it to be portrayed (Moore *et al.*, 1998).

Our aim was to facilitate the sharing of ideas about ways of improving support, and to set in place concrete plans for making sure that changes would begin to happen. One week before the workshop day, a 'drop-in day' was held to enable prospective participants to come and familiarise themselves with the chosen venue and to ask any questions they might have about what would be happening. The drop-in day was intended to reinforce the message that the workshops would be for families, and to alleviate any apprehensions about what was planned. It proved an extremely useful strategy for establishing confidence for working together with service providers and was, we feel, a key determinant of the success of the subsequent workshop which had a significant impact in the focal community.

The initial part of the programme was intended to clarify the priorities of people with learning difficulties, their older caregivers and practitioners. Participants worked in role-defined groups so they were able to focus specifically on the issues which were important to them. These role-defined workshops were then followed by a feedback session at which a representative of each group could relay what they had been discussing to the other groups. To get the discussion off to a lively start, the first workshops looked at some of the things that make service providers and families angry. We then moved on to ideas for overcoming some of the difficulties which were being recognised, and for dismantling barriers which participants perceived to be impeding service delivery. The final part of the programme involved each individual caregiver and service provider drawing up a practical plan of immediate action which they could realistically take to bring about some sort of tangible improvement in their situation over the next 3 months.

Participants with learning difficulties were facilitated in their group explorations by the involvement of advocates. Discussion focused around 3 main themes:

1. *'things we are good at'*
   – *to elicit skills for ordinary living;*
2. *'things we don't like'*
   – *to find out life-style preferences;*
3. *'what we would like to do with our lives'*
   – *to identify areas for possible change.*

Action plans were not formulated by participants with learning difficulties: instead, their contributions were summarised in picture-based reports of their explorations which were then widely circulated.

Many changes in service provision were mooted during the day and translated into plans for immediate action. For example, a group of practitioners pledged to develop an information leaflet to clarify their roles, responsibilities and powers to address confusion about who does what within providing agencies. A group of caregivers derived a plan for creating opportunities for them to meet jointly with the staff of a local, respite care hostel. Other action plans covered finding better ways of letting caregivers know about alternative care arrangements, holding accessible information sessions and improving responses to emergencies.

The workshop gave one caregiver a rare opportunity to talk at length to providers about the difficulties of making links with professionals who would respond at any given moment. As a result, she was delighted to receive a list of all social workers and community nurses in her area. However, several months after receiving the list, she still did not know who was who; she simply had information giving names. She pointed out 'the biggest problem is never getting to know the faces behind the names'. This provides a good example of how even the smallest individual action can bring about important change. It is very easy for service providers to make sure that whoever they are talking to does know their name, especially if there are frequent changes of staff. Information is an essential ingredient of citizenship: not least, very basic information, such as what people like to be called. Without information, people are unable to pursue their entitlements. The importance of providing information at many levels, and in accessible formats for everyone to whom it is relevant, must not be underestimated.

Bringing caregivers, people with learning difficulties and practitioners face to face, made visible many factors which could contribute to a strong sense of practitioner direction and a feeling of mutual support. During the proceedings, it was important to ensure that everyone could make contributions and feel positive about themselves and about the group. We found a great deal was achieved by involving a range of stakeholders in the course of a sustained interaction, in which they shared a relationship of interdependence, in the pursuit of common goals.

> We need more meetings and discussions of our ideas.
> [We need to] exchange feelings, problems and views
> and supporting ideas for the comfort and future of
> our disabled loved ones.

Practitioners agreed that this should happen more often and welcomed the chance to hear the views of carers, described by one caregiver as a much needed opportunity for 'telling people what makes me frustrated and about what I do'. There were real and tangible outcomes as a letter from one caregiver shows:

> *I have been into [the respite care hostel] and we have made arrangements for a coffee morning ... the officer in charge of the hostel was delighted with the idea and suggested he invited social services along. He said he would have lots of points to put forward to the carers of his own ideas. He welcomed the idea very much. Letters will be going out soon. This is an opportunity for all carers to meet the staff.*

Responses to a similar attempt to break down the perceived distance between caregivers and staff in a Day Centre were, however, very different:

> *Been into the Training Centre. They saw quite a few problems regarding a coffee morning. But to leave the idea with her. Some of the clients work at the Centre and [the Centre Manager] wants as little upset as possible. She was quite sure she could come up with something – maybe about six parents or carers at a time so as not to disrupt the arrangements of their day... Will chase up if nothing happens.*

Low expectations of service providers are clear from the remark *'will chase up if nothing happens'*. The situation is complicated because staff at the centre are accountable to people with learning difficulties first and *not* their caregivers. But this seems a classic example of where partnership initiatives could probably produce benefits for all parties. It is, anyway, plain that the interests of service users are structured around the preferences of service providers in the above response. Of course, professionals working for people with learning difficulties have the power to exclude caregivers from collaboration if they so wish. There will be situations where agreement about involving caregivers cannot easily be ascertained; for example, where people with learning difficulties have experienced abuse within their family, practitioners may feel caregivers have placed themselves beyond the 'decent' boundaries for partnership. But for the majority of families, which we have found are reputable and sincere, there are caregivers who would like to work collaboratively with providers of learning disability services and our evidence suggests much mutual gain is likely to come from viewing boundaries generously. Otherwise, the concerns of caregivers are trivialised and practitioners run the risk of alienating key allies.

EARNING TRUST

> *Who can I trust? It is so important to develop partnerships with the local authority, with the health authority, with the voluntary organisations, but it is difficult to know who you can trust. I trust my family and I trust other people who have had the same sort of problems through their life as I have had. So I trust parents, not professionals. History has taught me that.*

The issue of trust seems to be the key to whether caregivers and people with learning difficulties will talk openly to practitioners, particularly about long-term plans. It is worth reminding ourselves of how extensive the damage which stems from losing trust can be. The mother quoted below vividly recalled the first time professionals had shaken her trust, over thirty years ago:

> *The first time he went into short-term care he was eight months old, and he went into hospital and he was beautiful when he went in. He was the most bonniest baby you've ever seen and he came out like a real washed-out Down's Syndrome. He'd lost weight and I was worried.*
> *I went to the doctor and he said 'you'll have to get used to it'.*

There has to be trust between practitioners, caregivers and people with learning difficulties before plans for the future, and ways in which families and providing agencies might work together, can begin to be explored. Trust has to be earned. Outcomes from the joint workshop and subsequent meetings quickly made user participants much less wary of practitioners and allowed practitioners to be less anxious about user expectations. Joint discussions help show that practitioners are themselves aware of possible shortcomings and affirm their commitment to doing better; caregivers and people with learning difficulties say these acknowledgements help win their confidence.

MAKING HEADWAY THROUGH ACKNOWLEDGING BARRIERS

Our project workshops undoubtedly unleashed many contentious and difficult issues for practitioners. Some of the discussions raised questions of human and civil rights and point to substantial changes at the level of practitioner involvement, purchasing agency and policy-making. Nevertheless, those who participated showed themselves prepared to offer significant support for these changes. An important starting point has been in the personal reflection and reconceptualisation that those who attended the research workshops were prepared to make. Many existing barriers to the support aspirations of caregivers and their sons and daughters with learning difficulties, were dismantled as a consequence.

Some practitioners, for example, took immediate steps to enable caregivers to present their ideas for the future to Social Services. These included arrangements where parents move out from the home and their son or daughter stays with co-residents or support staff as required, which would, for some people, amount to having their dreams come true. Participating families have received, and expressed appreciation of, reassurances that providers share their aspiration for people with learning difficulties to be established in their different circumstances before a crisis ensues. There has been special recognition of the fact that all members of the family are keen to ensure that co-residents or support staff are suitable for, and compatible with the person with learning difficulties. Participating providers have reaffirmed their commitment to keep talking to families.

The pursuit of the ideal should not be forgotten and the small steps of the realistic need to be placed within this greater framework. However, it is important not to undermine the very tangible benefits that can be brought about through modest changes. Provider and user participants involved in this project started to make a real and valued difference to the situation of caregivers and people with learning difficulties by carrying out action plans that were *jointly* developed.

Accepting that there is pressure on resources leads many people to abandon their real aspirations for support and to resign themselves to the notion that any sort of assistance, however minor or ill-adapted to their needs, is something to be grateful for. This 'fact of life' syndrome clearly constitutes a source of disempowerment for families. Barriers to shared planning are commonplace. One caregiver heard about the closure of a respite care home her son regularly used through the local newspaper. People feel reluctant to complain as they suspect this might cause services to be taken away from them. Little wonder then that looking into the future can be a daunting task, not least, where people are aware of or do not feel in control of possible options.

> *We want to complain, but we don't know what to complain about, and how to complain*

Caregivers and people with learning difficulties frequently find themselves without knowledge of how to criticise the way services are run and with little motivation to assert their rights to services which, the Carers (Recognition and Services) Act states, they are entitled (Carers National Association 1996). The Act itself gives caregivers the right to ask for an assessment of their ability to provide or to continue to provide care, but a report by the Carers National Association (1997) revealed that only eighteen per cent of caregivers surveyed had asked for an assessment. Of those not asking, fifty-three per cent had not been informed of their rights to have an assessment, forty-nine per cent did not know how an assessment could help them and thirty-eight per cent did not know they were entitled to an assessment. For those who had an assessment, the outcomes have reportedly been positive; sixty-nine per cent were offered services, fifty-five per cent had their services increased and fifty-nine per cent expressed satisfaction with the outcomes of the assessment. If entitlements are to make any real impact, practitioners must be vigilant about checking that people are aware of what is on offer and know how to get it. This is not a simple matter. Families also need to know how to challenge decisions and use complaints procedures and going through these processes with a sympathetic, well-informed practitioner can help to evolve improved practice (McDonald, 1999).

LOOKING TO THE FUTURE

Many people are uncertain about specifying what support they would like because experience has taught them to expect very little and to manage on their own. Yet we know that caregivers are supporting people with learning difficulties in the context of loving and protective family relationships and are quite clear about what areas of concern lay ahead. What they want is for their concerns to be acknowledged by providing agencies. Often this simply involves creative responses within the framework of what is already on offer. Gains can be made through acknowledging resource constraints which means that suspicions that decisions are entirely budget-led can be reduced.

> People with learning difficulties and their caregivers are 'not greedy; nor are they looking to abandon their relatives at the first opportunity. They merely want peace of mind for the present and for the future. Is that too much to ask?'
>
> **(Walker and Walker, 1998)**

Dreams and budgets *can* be reconciled given a resolute approach to maximising choice and to creating new precedents when called for.

Rethinking common obstacles

ACKNOWLEDGING ASPIRATIONS

> *I hope to be included in my sons' lives as long as I'm alive.*

Wherever possible, initiatives should be developed to raise the standard of consultation by genuinely enabling caregivers to play an active role in decisions about the future of their family. Where people are partners in procedures identifying their needs, and in planning how they will be met, a great deal of needless worry can be alleviated. Typical concerns expressed by caregivers give an illustration:

> *I don't know whether a carer stays in overnight or what they do if anything happens in the night, but that's the sort of thing we want for Sandra. She doesn't like being by herself.*
>
> *[ideally] it will be staffed by – you know – fully trained people and they will have night people there as well because John needs twenty-four hour care.*
>
> *Luke Jones [a person who moved away from living with older caregivers to an independent situation] he had his flat door on fire didn't he? Now there's only one door on them flats. He had a chip pan fire you know.*

Not knowing whether your son or daughter is safe at night or at risk from fire are likely to be huge sources of anxiety for the majority of parents at any time of life. The quotes above make plain how removing the tyranny of 'otherness' when thinking around older caregivers and people with learning difficulties can transform planning. Once such anxieties are brought home in the minds of practitioners, they can start to be properly acknowledged, and emphasis can be placed on bringing about feasible solutions.

ASSURANCES ABOUT THE QUALITY OF SUPPORT

Assurances about the quality of support that will be made available to people with learning difficulties when, or if, they enter into new lifestyles need to be backed up by clear preparatory action. If one family can endorse the support that their son or daughter receives to another family contemplating change, then the path of new arrangements is clearly much smoother. Respect for the viewpoint of caregivers is vital. Often, caregivers focus their struggle on the bare minimum of entitlements, saying, for example

'I would want to be able to walk in and help with the washing up. Help with seeing Michael off to the centre, you know, as long as I could ... or just go and sit with him'.

But a lack of prior experience of involvement on decision-making has left many dubious about having their right to a say respected. As part of improving communication and partnership, it will be important to create safe forums in which people can express different views and conflicting priorities. Arrangements for dealing with disputes, and information about these, need to be expanded where practitioners are serious about building on the views of caregivers and people with learning difficulties.

An immediate strategy, designed to ensure that provision is appropriate and valued, **is to identify aspirations – and then possibilities *not* the other way round**.

It is important to create confidence in personal choice and control. A persistent negative consequence of overlooking aspirations is the creation of unnecessary anxiety. For example, caregivers using respite facilities for the first time might benefit from sharing their views of their relatives' ideal bedtime, their food preferences, what they like to wear, and so on. One family desperately wanted to share information about their traditions for

opening birthday cards and presents so that they could
feel sure their daughter would recognise her special day.

> *I was delighted with the new arrangements for respite
> care. Every three months I am being asked by phone for
> my dates for short respite care for the next three months.
> They also confirm by telephone and by letter. There
> has been a big improvement since twelve months ago.*

SHARED DECISION-MAKING

We often find that caregivers do not receive information
about arrangements concerning their sons or daughters.
This reinforces fear and creates barriers if they believe this
is indicative of what would happen if the person with
learning difficulties moved out of the family home. One of
the most common anxieties we uncovered is that contact
will be reduced and attachments eroded if people with
learning difficulties move away from their older caregivers.
This is not unfounded as one person described:

> *I went into the centre to see him one Monday and they
> said* 'Oh he's not here' *so I said* 'Why? Where is he?'
> 'Oh he's poorly'.
> *I said* 'Why didn't anybody tell me?'
> *So I went straight to the phone in the special care
> room, phoned and said* 'When was John taken ill?'
> *So they said* 'He wasn't well when he came home on
> Friday afternoon so we called the doctor out Friday
> night.'
> *I said* 'Why on earth didn't you tell me?' *The whole
> weekend and this poor lad with all these strangers
> around him and Mum wasn't there.*

The inner pain of proposed or actual separation does not
need to be imagined – it is familiar from our own experiences
of life. There were many long-lasting consequences for
John and his family in terms of growing doubt that service
providers could be trusted to make adequate
arrangements for the separate lives of family members. We
must demonstrate real commitment to upholding the

rights of people to have contact with significant family members and friends if heartache is to be avoided.

Increasing time for shared decision-making is emotionally supportive, helps establish mutual trust, brings a sense of purpose to interactions between caregivers, people with learning difficulties and practitioners and leads to coherent and valued outcomes. Any assault on trust reinforces negative perceptions.

MAKING SENSE OF RESISTANCE TO ADVICE ABOUT CHANGE

A common fear, which stems from a lack of participation in discussions with practitioners, is that caregivers, and older caregivers in particular, feel themselves to be under threat of losing their entitlement to continue supporting the person with learning difficulties. Some consideration needs to be given to this as complex interests are involved and sensitivity is called for.

> *[If service providers think I can't cope] they'll take him off me and no way will I have him. You see, once you let go of them and let them go, you have nothing whatsoever to do with them. You can go and visit, but you're not his guardian any more. They are his guardian. They can move him wherever they want and I can't do a thing about it.*

We may forget that caregivers are parents first. Stereotypes of caregivers as potentially buckling under enormous strains, as over-protective, unfamiliar with new trends and so on pathologise those who support people with learning difficulties. Caregivers are painfully aware of this and often feel themselves under surveillance. In this way, they are routinely disempowered and express worries about being condemned as bad parents – a hapless and patronising phrase, commonly heard, is 'parents reluctant to let go'.

Assurances that 'mother knows best' are withdrawn from older caregivers, and professionals can unknowingly position themselves as experts with 'newer' or 'better' knowledge about what is best for people with learning difficulties, frequently making judgement with reference to concepts which are not part of a family's discourse –

including 'advocacy', 'empowerment' and 'autonomy.' This can be detected in the characteristic disquiet expressed by a practitioner we interviewed about an older caregiver questioning the value of self-advocacy:

> *We have a client who has joined a self advocacy group, whose Mum is quite protective and orders him about basically in his life. And one night she came in from being out all day working and was very tired and said to him* 'Oh just pass that over please' *which was a footstool and he said* 'Well you know where it is' *and he would never have done that. She was unhappy that the advocacy service was teaching her son, because she felt that she was losing control of him.*

There is no concession to the different emphasis which people in divergent roles necessarily (and rightly) place on theories which, after all, most older caregivers have seen come and go in various guises during the course of their caregiving career. Even if practitioners object to the reactions of caregivers to encounters with new approaches, it is obvious that the meanings attached to changes will profoundly influence the way in which those changes impact on family life. It is to be expected that the impact of self-advocacy, for example, will be complicated and affect caregivers in many different ways. It seems important to ensure that professionals are well equipped to support caregivers struggling with notions they may well perceive to be relatively new and untried. Understanding why caregivers may view change with a pinch of salt involves respecting their long experience of parenting. It is also worth acknowledging that practitioners too sometimes perceive change as threatening. New initiatives may radically improve people's lives, but there can be counter-productive offshoots.

> *Mrs. B.: What's advocacy?*
> *Mrs. E.: Thinking for yourself.*
> *Mrs. B.: Why the hell don't they say so? I mean, why put those damn great words in?*
> **(Cited in Sutcliffe and Simons 1993, p. 92)**

Caregivers may well fear repercussions if they fail to adopt new ways, which practitioners favour yet with which they are uncomfortable. Practitioners supporting people with learning difficulties are not compelled to take the opinions of caregivers into account and those supporting older people may not feel it appropriate to focus on their adult children. Closer integration of services may be necessary. All of this needs further examination. Key questions to explore are:

- When does the right to be autonomous and self-directed in your parenting stop?
- What rights do caregivers have to resist advice, particularly to resist advice on behalf of an adult with learning difficulties?
- What happens when the rights of caregivers and those of people with learning difficulties they support are at odds?
- What is the status of a caregiver's knowledge and how is this weighed in relation to the knowledge of an adult who has learning difficulties and in relation to the knowledge practitioners have?

We frequently uncover 'caregiver blaming' discourses, such as that a person with learning difficulties is unduly influenced by a parent. These give rise to standpoints which allow the wider role of social influences on the situation of people with learning difficulties to be ignored (including the potentially inadequate impact one is presumably making oneself when such a discourse unfolds). There are several observations which may prompt practitioners to see things more clearly from an older caregiver's perspective:

- Caregivers are frequently pathologised as parents.
- Older people do not fit with particular cultural ideas about fitness for caregiving.
- Older caregivers are expected to engage with advice about care of people with learning difficulties when they are not at an age which fits the usual picture of people on the receiving end of advice about their sons or daughters. This compromises their credibility: when they are the focus of

◄   public debate, they fall outside both the domain of credible caregivers – 'they are getting too old', and the domain of credible parents – 'they are too fixed in their ways to know what is best'.

●   Those in the position of bestowing advice may not have experience of parenting or they may well be similar in age to the person whose life is being discussed. While such factors are not inevitably associated with unsatisfactory practice, if caregivers feel inappropriately judged, relations may be strained.

Practitioners are increasingly comfortable arguing that parents are the experts when talking about their infants and young children, but they dispute this when talking about older parents who continue in their role as primary caregivers. It is inadmissible that the wishes of people with learning difficulties should be swamped by the views of anyone else when it comes to future planning, but when conflict is created through suppressing the voice of caregivers then outcomes are likely to be in some jeopardy.

It is easy to undermine the status of a caregiver's knowledge. Their knowledge is rooted in experiential knowledge of living with a particular individual in a particular situation and so can be dismissed as 'too subjective'. Their views can quite easily be implicitly (or explicitly) criticised by referring to professional information which can be inflated through references to academic knowledge and claimed as more substantially *known*. It is not then surprising that some older caregivers adopt a position of resistance to advice. They can point out that *'the theories are always changing' – 'they used to say this and now they say this'* – and their confidence in professional guidance is undermined (Alldred, 1996). These points bring together a variety of tensions for practitioners seeking to support caregivers and people with learning difficulties:

●   there are competing agendas;
●   these agendas need acknowledging;
●   competing agendas need reconciling – not domination of one over the other.

Read (2000) provides many useful insights into these issues from her research on listening to mother.

An adequate approach needs to recognise not only the quality of life for the individual service users but the added quality of life issues which are implicated for those with whom they live. Practitioners who work hard to consolidate a genuine feeling of respect for the people they are involved with are the most enabling. Looking afresh at frequently encountered sticking points can suggest worthwhile avenues for change. We need to try to view caregivers and people with learning difficulties in terms which we would find acceptable if applied to ourselves.

Implementing change

Most caregivers wish to see the adjustment of their loved one to new living arrangements take place in their lifetime. They know change may bring many advantages including, perhaps, increased quality time spent together but they struggle with feelings of love and loyalty and not wanting to upset their sons or daughters through instigating change.

On the other hand, there are times when people with learning difficulties wish to pursue an independent life before their caregivers feel ready. In any event, families need to be able to explore future living options slowly and they place emphasis on flexibility and being able to backtrack if things do not work out. They do not want to feel that their family relationships are being contested when it comes to changing living arrangements.

> *It would also be a great comfort to the family to know that she's [going to be] experiencing independence, but at the same time she's in good hands and they don't have to worry.*
>
> *She needs to experience some independence ... with being around parents who know her situation, she's not able to obtain that confidence.*

PLANNED AND WELL-PREPARED CHANGE

> *We want to know **at this stage** what's going to happen to him when we pop off you see. He could settle down in a flat or in a house with two or three other people, I'm sure ... but how would anybody go about it supposing we pop off? He wouldn't know the first thing about who to apply to.*
>
> *I don't know what is in the future, what arrangements social services are making for the future, I don't know.*

The prospect of unplanned or ill-prepared change is a major stress factor. People are fearful of temporary arrangements and frequent changes. Above all, they worry about the person with learning difficulties losing the possibility of one day returning home or trying new options if things do not work out. Conceivable reasons for this include unsuitable workers or staff hostility or not getting on with new living partners. What is needed are transitional arrangements which are reversible and which recognise that people change their minds, that sometimes things do not turn out as we hope, that homesickness is a reality when people first find themselves without day-to-day family support, and that life is generally unpredictable. Infrequent contact, or the possibility of contact breaking down entirely, are real concerns which often come down to practical matters for practitioners.

What I want for the future for him is a home he can get to know as his second home but not to be in it permanently to begin with. I don't want to lose him, you see, until the time comes.

It would be lovely if he could stay there for a few days a week and just perhaps come home at weekends.

I would like a social worker to visit pretty often. You know, to come and see whether the heating was all right or not … a visitor, you know, 2 or 3 times a week, just to see that everything was all right with him …

Much effective support can be gained when practitioners find out where distances, transport and costs might prove problematic and take steps to circumvent these. It could come down to very simple matters such as finding out a bus route or details of ticket concessions. Caregivers and people with learning difficulties feel that the chances of new living arrangements succeeding are much improved if they can be assured of continued contact, with flexible contact arrangements put firmly in place before changes are made. They know that their paths may not neatly intersect once the family no longer lives together as a unit, but they want to tighten up the possibilities.

EXPLAINING SYSTEMS

> *They come and they go, you get a different name every time you ring up, the last time I rang up for this Jane Wood. 'Oh, I'm sorry, she's left'. I said 'who do I speak to?' ... And you're speaking again to someone you don't know, again.*

There are practical obstacles that everybody encounters which necessitate practitioners developing systems that enable tensions to be reduced. Frequent staff changes may be a fact of life but they also make life very difficult unless expedient contingency plans for ensuring continuity have been put in place. Improved consultation when passing over caseloads would enable smoother transitions. In addition, service users feel that practitioners miss out on valuable information by not consulting with them when reorganisation is proposed. Personnel continually changing is a very real problem. However, this is very much a concern for social workers too, who fear they will not be allowed space or time to complete activities which are often seen, organisationally, as relatively low priority. Unquestionably, this is a management issue and service providers and service users might profitably work together to fight for improvements in this corner.

> *Interviewer: And you don't have a social worker or anything like that?*
> *Respondent: No*
> *Interviewer: Would you like one?*
> *Respondent: No. Not while I can manage.*

Few caregivers and people with learning difficulties in our study had regular contact with a care manager: many did not know who they were. People sometimes decide to 'go it alone' in despair following unsatisfactory experience of support. Others are left alone by default: *'I haven't got a social worker, you know. They don't rush themselves at all'.*

> *I like social workers to stay in the job longer and they get used to you and you can get used to them, but they don't stay ... they are always leaving, chopping and changing, that's what worries me over Tom in years to come. You know, all this that they've got wrote down, and the people that are there now, who will be there when Tom needs them?*

These remarks hint at a common confusion. It is fairly typical to find that people have not had the difference between the current system of care management and a former system of social worker allocation, which they may have known for years, properly explained to them:

> *People used to have an allocated social worker who would work to support their interests on an ongoing basis. However, it was felt social workers were consequently carrying too big a caseload and the Care Management system was brought in. Care managers take on a referral and work with the individual until the aim of the referral has been achieved and a care plan has been drawn up. The 'case' then closes.*
>
> *So, for example, I could put in a referral for an individual who has little to do during the day. A care manager would pick up the referral and start work with the individual person on the particulars of their referral. When this work is done, and an outcome is arrived at, the care manager closes the case. If another referral for the same individual is put in regarding another issue, it may be picked up by the same care manager but is equally likely to be picked up by someone else.*
>
> **Family Support Worker's comments**

The way things are organised may need careful explanation.

A practice pointer posed by Booth and Booth (1994) calls for practitioners to

> *be aware of the capacity for exacerbating the stress on families and augmenting the problems they face.*
> **(Booth and Booth, 1994, p. 149)**

As each family goes through a range of interactions and outcomes over the years, let-downs or perceived inconsistencies can create scepticism and make it likely that provider – user relationships will *generally* be viewed with distrust:

> *you're dealing with people who you've never set eyes on saying* 'Well, can't Melanie do this? And can't Melanie do that?'
> *I wouldn't be asking if Melanie could do it'.*

Families are realistic. They recognise that many professionals do not enjoy conditions of service that encourage them to stay in any one position for long. They do not imagine that a quick solution to this problem is available, but emphasise the degree of difficulty which this brings. Some feel it is assumed that other family members will help out with support, when in fact this is not always the case:

> *I didn't think I need worry because I had such a large family and I thought perhaps each would take it in turns to have [my son], but I was wrong and they don't want him.*

> *They are kind of juggling their workers around ... I haven't met this latest one, but I'm now on my third agency and each time I'm hoping that this is going to be it and I'm going to actually get somebody who will be able to cope with Shaun and bath him, and that I will be able to just relax.*

- What are the best ways of getting across information about how services are organised?
- What is the value of meeting with people with learning difficulties and caregivers when relationships are new?
- What practical steps can be taken to achieve better continuity of support, particularly when the time available is constrained or changes are unexpected?

OBSTACLES TO PLANNING

Discussing future support is undoubtedly difficult and emotionally charged. Many people find it a particularly upsetting and worrying business:

you know, if anything happened to us ... no, I don't like to think about it,

I was a bit of an ostrich.

But the reasons for discomfort are not simple. Reluctance to talk about the future is not wholly explained, as might be supposed, by reluctance to face up to one's own mortality or the prospective death of a child. There are important questions to ask about what else parents might be fearful of, because this very often turns out to be things that practitioners can quite easily deal with.

We repeatedly find people dwelling on fears which a shared understanding of the principles of community care planning could take away. Some, for example, will not know that emphasis should be routinely placed on independent living outcomes wherever possible. If practitioners do not make this explicit then people may be, and often are, troubled by outdated impressions that residential care is the only option and they will have no choice or control. The years during which many families try to avoid thinking about the future could be freed up for planning and developing confidence about future options if practitioners can show readiness to discover what the blocks to planning are. Janet's fear –

'I didn't want him to have to go into a home. And my husband was very, very, very much against him going

into a home'
– reminds us that the movement for independent living may
be well ingrained in the minds of practitioners but it cannot
be assumed that the concept is equally familiar to service
users.

There seems to be a critical, albeit difficult, role for service
providers as enablers of planning processes. Fear of the
unknown plays a large part in refusal to acknowledge what
might happen next. In this sense, service providers are just as
vulnerable as service users. Acknowledging concerns is likely
to give a useful starting point from which to commence
reducing uncertainty. If families can hold on to the
expectation that providing agencies will at least acknowledge
their dreams and pay attention to their nightmares, then they
might begin to be less reluctant to think about some of the
things they ordinarily dread bringing to the front of their
minds. All of this reaffirms the need for practitioners to:

- take the time to become accustomed to a families' hopes and
  fears;
- examine one's own role in any delayed decision-making.

In some cases, repeated discussions will be necessary, as
not all of the possibilities can be explored at once, families
may change their minds and circumstances alter. Even if
explorations are time-consuming and plans seem
uncertain or idealistic, the investment of respect for the
families priorities will help circumvent many barriers to
good communications in the years ahead.

*Why do service providers, especially local authority
providers, speak a different language?*

A tip from caregivers for anyone anxious about mooting
discussions about the future and possible separations: *'be
straightforward.'* Avoid the confusion, bewilderment and
sometimes resentment, which can be built out of a more
cautious approach. People are more likely to be crushed
by speculation and imagined fears than by frank discussion
and appraisal.

FATAL CONSEQUENCES OF INADEQUATE RESPONSES

I've heard a lot of women say this, 'I'm not really afraid
to die but I don't want to, while my son or my
handicapped daughter is still alive'. *And a lot of them
say that they are thinking of taking them with them
when they go. You know, overdosing them.*

At a public lecture, Michael Oliver reminded the audience
that complacency about disabled people's lives has death-
making consequences (Oliver, 1999). Our research has
thrown up disturbing evidence that confirms this. We find
that euthanasia is an outcome firmly fixed in the minds of
many of those with older caregiving responsibilities. In
our view, this is a direct result of the failure of those
involved in community care to respond to the demands of
people with learning difficulties and their caregivers
adequately. We have, however, found it extremely difficult
to get taken seriously the death-making consequences of a
disregard for the entitlements of these two groups of
people.

There is a great deal of denial around the possibility
that failures of community care can have fatal
consequences. For example, the topic emerged at a
meeting of a major UK agency concerned with people
with learning difficulties and their older caregivers, which
was attended by many of the key players shaping policy
and practice in this area. One participant dismissed
uneasiness about euthanasia on the grounds that
quantitative research does not indicate that it is a
concern. The dismissal was hotly contested. Many of those
present said that they knew people who were
contemplating euthanasia. The point was made that
quantitative research invariably reduces the views of
caregivers to fit a set of categories shaped around the
interests of researchers. Questionnaire data, for example,
has simply regulated and reproduced existing ways in
which the experiences and viewpoints of caregivers have
been described. There was a strong argument that, when
given the opportunity to talk at length and on their own
terms, people are much more likely to be forthcoming

about intimate and distressing issues in their lives. This discussion dominated a large part of the proceedings yet was completely dropped from the minutes of the meeting – rendering contemplated euthanasia invisible and closing off the possibility of further debate in an influential forum.

Clearly, there is a substantial problem. Research projects provide a crucial route through which serious social problems should be identified. If researchers themselves collude in the concealment of those problems then the relevance of our research, and our integrity as researchers, becomes highly questionable. There is a key role for practitioners to play in insisting that research is open and rigorous and that it makes connections to the deepest levels of need which they and their clients are witnessing.

The comments of caregivers in our research and support work are not fiction. Yet the fatal consequences of failings in community care are frequently – and, we have found, formally and institutionally – swept under the carpet, even within some of the leading agencies which claim to support caregivers and people with learning difficulties. There is no doubt, that in families which have no confidence in practitioner support, death-making arrangements are felt to be preferable to entrusting a much loved person with learning difficulties to community care providers. Some caregivers actively seek the right to take this course of action:

> *You've got to accept the situation; you've got to make sure that you put pressure on your MPs and so on, and make sure that you elect people who are in favour of euthanasia; that's an absolute certainty.*

Some disabled people go through with ending their own lives – as we found through our association with the death of a person who so distrusted the capacity of social services to provide acceptable long-term support that they opted for suicide by starvation. There is an urgent need identified here to raise expectations for disabled people and for caregivers. The whole community, and not just service providers, can no longer shy away from questions about euthanasia.

It is imperative for practitioners to think about the individual and collective action they can take in immediate response to these monumental issues. The acute fact facing service providers here is that disabled people are under threat for their very existence if they and their caregivers cannot expect, and be given, more tangible support in their struggle for control over their future affairs. Ambivalence from professionals towards the fatal consequences of service failures, in contexts where people feel there are no adequate provisions for the long-term future, unequivocally reinforces vulnerability. We are not suggesting that professionals intentionally dismiss the euthanasia discourse but the reality of alternatives to best practice have to be faced. Is it possible to be proactive and arrange a seminar to discuss these issues? How *laissez-faire* can we be?

Caregivers often tell us that they do not know how to safeguard the future of their sons or daughters with learning difficulties. Where practitioners have provided practical help with the business of making wills and setting up funding arrangements, families have gained considerable peace of mind. This is an example of a practical strategy that can increase confidence in the future and help carve out options other than euthanasia.

WILLS AND TRUSTS

Knowing how to make a will ... insurance policies ... a lot of people won't insure our children. I have to do it through Mencap and insure my son through them because his funeral will cost just as much as for anybody else.

Making a will can ensure that caregivers protect the future of the person with learning difficulties with whom they are concerned. There are a number of issues that need thinking through when planning to leave money or possessions to a son or daughter, such as preserving their right to benefits, securing future accommodation and drawing up the *right* will. What may be of greatest

importance is how to get information, advice and
guidance on legal issues that is specifically geared to both
probate law and to the interests of people with learning
difficulties.

There is an Association of Lawyers for People with
Learning Difficulty in the UK which anyone can access.
Voluntary agencies also have useful legal departments and
can advise on innovations such as the Mencap Trusteeship
Scheme through which caregivers can appoint someone to
look out for the future interests of a person with learning
difficulties.

*Discretionary Trusts are, on the whole, the main
way to protect your [son's or daughter's] financial
future, and are one way of ensuring that they receive
their inheritance without affecting state benefits, as
the Trust fund is not taken into account by the DSS for
the assessment of income support. Such a trust
involves putting the inheritance in the hands of
trustees, who are then responsible for using the
inheritance in the interests of the person with learning
difficulties.*

*You appoint the trustees. It is important that the
trustees know the person with learning disabilities, as
they can then be sure that money is being spent as he
or she would wish. Consequently family and friends
are common choices. It is usually better to have two
trustees, one who knows the individual well and
another who can take care of the accounts. Because of
this it might be useful to appoint a professional such
as a solicitor as one of the trustees, although they will
usually make a charge.*

**(From *Sorting Out The Future*, a leaflet
produced by Central & South Manchester MENCAP
and The Manchester Joint Service for People
with Learning Disabilities)**

A critical and much neglected question is how to support
people with learning difficulties in making their own wills.
Some voluntary agencies are just beginning to evolve
forums for enabling people with learning difficulties to do

this. When people with learning difficulties are placed in the position of prospective will-makers, and not simply regarded as the passive recipients of other people's provisions, the impact on the planning of their future is likely to be transforming, not only for themselves, but for their caregivers, their wider family and the community beyond.

The role of a will is primarily to pull together the central elements of what one hopes to lay down in the future. When people are unable to consolidate their plans in this way their futures are riddled with uncertainty.

- What changes can be implemented in your own work setting that would make confidence in the future achievable?

Listening differently

WHAT DO PEOPLE WITH LEARNING DIFFICULTIES WANT?
**Much of the data on which this book is based was
collected under the auspices of local social services
and health authority providers. The fact that none of
the participating caregivers, people with learning
difficulties or service providers went so far as to
challenge the existence and power of these agencies
may be a consequence of this.**
It may be that the self-advocacy movement will, in time to
come, generate more radical options than those posed by
our analysis. These points have been made elsewhere by
people with learning difficulties who wish to stress that
the pursuit of realistic change is not necessarily the pursuit
of their ideal future (Aspis, 1997). People with learning
difficulties are keen to extend the agenda, to focus not
simply on care in the future and where they will live, but
to stimulate broader considerations at the same time of
what kind of a future they might wish to have.

ASSUMPTIONS AROUND WHO GIVES CARE

> *I know he loves me and I know he knows that I love
> him ... sometimes when you're very down and feel
> very lonely, if an arm just comes round your shoulder,
> you get hugged ... Shaun does that and I know that it
> is all worthwhile.*

People with learning difficulties want recognition that the
caregiving relationship is not all one-sided. They give
companionship, love and care to their families, as well as
being recipients of care. And many caregivers stress the
value they place on what people with learning difficulties
bring to their lives.

> *Richard is thirty and lives with his mother and father.*
> *Both parents are older people and have developed*
> *chronic illnesses. Over the years Richard has taken on*
> *more responsibilities, including making drinks and*
> *helping with meals, cleaning the house and going to*
> *the shops. Richard also provides his parents with*
> *companionship and personal support when they need*
> *it.*
> *Richard's mother has made sure that Richard has*
> *plenty to do during the day and evening by*
> *arranging college courses and various evening groups*
> *which he regularly attends. She also makes sure that*
> *he gets to and from places and that his health needs*
> *are being met.*
>
> **Family support worker, Mencap**

Richard's situation above shows that it is a mistake to take the dependency of people with learning difficulties as given. Community care policy however, perpetuates focus on Richard as the recipient of care and effectively positions him as 'the problem'. It threatens to prevent practitioners from seeing any concerns which the family may face as a social phenomenon and thus we see the disabling consequences of prevalent discourses of dependency. The changing needs of caregivers, and the changing capabilities of people with learning difficulties, are eclipsed if practitioners fix their focus on people with learning difficulties as dependent.

Richard's family situation is typical of many which push at the edges of assumptions about who exactly the providers and recipients of care are when people with learning difficulties live with ageing parents. As parents get older, there are usually times when they would benefit from assistance or support. This is often provided by close family – commonly, sons and daughters and including those who have learning difficulties. This is not to suggest that people with learning difficulties inevitably find themselves providers of care to their ageing parents, but to highlight that as caregivers get older, in some circumstances, people with learning difficulties do routinely take on extra duties which constitute caregiving.

The point is that, while Richard's mother's care-giving is formally recognised, his is not.

It is almost universally presumed that people with learning difficulties are recipients of care and parents with whom they live are care providers. It is important for practitioners to examine assumptions about where the locus of responsibility for caregiving lies within a family. In Richard's family, which is far from unique, the relationship is reciprocal and there is mutual and shared recognition of difficulty and providing of support. When Tony Blair said *'we should take pride in carers'* (1999) it must be hoped that he included disabled people as providers of care in his thinking.

SELDOM-HEARD VOICES

People with learning difficulties have historically been denied the opportunity to engage in discussions which respect their adult status, and older caregivers are consequently pushed into trying to access and articulate their views for them. Practitioners may find that conversation with caregivers is easier and more comfortable than communication with people with learning difficulties. Nevertheless, it is crucial that means are found of enabling people with learning difficulties to speak for themselves. Sometimes, watching and observing can prove more insightful than talking and listening.

> *Lucy is continually distressed because staff in her residential accommodation get angry if she sits on the floor by a radiator as this blocks their way. Any practitioner who spent time observing Lucy at home with her parents before she moved would have known that*
> *(a) she likes to sit by radiators*
> *and*
> *(b) she likes to have a good view of what is going on. Is it unreasonable to think that a radiator might have been moved to suit?*
> **Therapist talking about her sister**

There are many difficult matters, particularly when a

system of communication relies on intermediaries.

The issue of mediating options for future living is not mooted in relation to adults without learning difficulties, and parents are not ordinarily afforded the right to influence the decisions of their adult children. Yet people with learning difficulties are regularly denied their right to consider future options for living at first hand. People with learning difficulties are often excluded from a meaningful role in consultation processes. At best, caregivers are positioned as quasi 'communication supporters', expected to facilitate dialogue with unfamiliar people.

Several points are worth making. First, caregivers can enable excellent access for people with learning difficulties to the planning process. Communication is facilitated through their familiarity with, and sensitivity to their son's or daughter's preferred interactive medium and language. On the other hand, however, both the person with learning difficulties and the practitioner have to trust the judgement and skill of the older caregiver who is positioned as communication facilitator and vice versa. Subtle changes of language and meaning can and do frequently occur and may be impossible to avoid. There is conspicuous powerlessness on all sides in such mediated interactions (Beazley *et al.*, 1997; Beazley 2000).

The third point is really an extension of the first two in terms of self-determination for people with learning difficulties. When communicating via third parties, practitioners have restricted access to disabled people's own articulations. Caregivers acting as communication facilitators may for one reason or another introduce shifts either linked to their own value systems and beliefs or in a desire to represent themselves or the person with learning difficulties in a certain light.

There is inevitably a level of dependency which will influence discussions and it is important for practitioners to be prepared for pitfalls when communication is indirect. Finally, there are hazards if either party wishes to discuss things which may unsettle relations either with the person with learning difficulties or with a caregiver or with providers. Practitioners will need to ask themselves:

- who needs to control discussions about future options for caregivers and people with learning difficulties to ensure they will generate outcomes in sympathy with each individual person's own agenda?
- to what extent are practitioners obliged to impose an agenda for self-expression and self-determination on people with learning difficulties who are not familiar with being asked to decide things for themselves and who, conceivably, may prefer their caregivers to decide things for them?
- how can practitioners access and reconcile the potentially different aspirations for future living arrangements held by people with learning difficulties and caregivers at the same time as being enabling and empowering to both parties?

There are no simple answers to these questions. Goodley (2000) describes how the stories of people with learning difficulties are a very useful medium through which to capture insider perspectives. We have also gained many invaluable insights into the preferences of people with learning difficulties through research which examines the role of performing arts as a vehicle for self expression (Moore and Goodley, 1999) which we draw on next to further the debate.

OPTIMISING REVIEWS

Practitioners will know that the main forum for bringing about change in the lives of people with learning difficulties is usually through the reviews process planning meeting attended by social workers, caregivers and other supporters such as key day-centre staff, in addition to the person with learning difficulties themselves. It is accepted in some areas that a helpful step in preparing for a 'reviews meeting' involves a trusted person exploring the views of the person with learning difficulties in advance of the meeting and making sure they know who will be present and why. However, deep dissatisfaction and sometimes resentment of reviews procedures has been uncovered time and time again in various of our research studies. People with learning difficulties are challenging complacency around reviews procedures through the performing arts. Their work identifies deficiencies in common practice and shows how things could be better.

A BAD REVIEW
(Description of a performance depicting a bad review lasting 3 minutes 35 seconds)

Paul: *The time is here, the place is now. We're going to show you how reviews should and shouldn't be.*

Three members of staff enter, a physiotherapist, a social worker and key worker, each introduced by Paul as he shows them to their seats.

Paul: *Is the first person ready to come in?*

The client, played by Kath, enters stage left with her mother Julie, who asks Kath if she is *'ready for this'*. Kath says *'yes'* and her mum tells her *'come on, let's get it over with'*. They sit down; Kath on one chair, her mother joining a chair at the end of the row of professionals. *'Oh, if you'll excuse me, I haven't got the right file'* says Paul. He leaves to get the right documents. He is away for a short while. Nothing is said in the room.

When he returns, Kath's mum asks if they can start.

'No' shouts Paul, turning from chairperson to the audience's story-teller.

'Now' he tells us, *'there are two people listening at the door who shouldn't be listening'*

Enter Alf, broom in hand, and Tina [stage right].

Alf: *What are you doing?*

Tina: *Shhh … I'm listening.*

'And there's two people in the Garden' points out Paul.

Enter Paula and Peter who appears to be looking into the room through binoculars [stage left].

Paula: *What's going on in there Peter?*

Peter: *There's an interview on.*   ▶

◀

'Now can we start', asks Kath's mother, impatiently. 'We may. Carry on', instructs Paul as he takes his seat in between the professionals with mother and Kath, sat on her own. The professionals talk among themselves.

Physio: *I hope this doesn't go on long.*

Social worker: [Tuts] *I have to go to another boring review.*

Mum: *OK. Can we start talking about [my daughter]?*

Physio: [To mother] *Well, [she] has been doing physio for the last 12 months and she's not really showing interest and she's finding it hard.*

Mother: *What is there exactly for her to do?*

Key worker: *Different courses, sewing, computers ...*

Social worker: *... caring for old people, child care.*

Mother: [Leaning over to physio] *Well, as her physio, what would you suggest?*

Physio: *Well ... she might find it difficult and things hard to do.*

Mother: *Well, this is it. She really can't do these things can she?*

Enter tea lady, *'I've brought a cup of tea'.*

Mother takes tea. Physio then stands telling his fellow staff and [client's] mother, that he has to go to another appointment. Shakes hands of staff and mum. Social and key worker follow suit. All leave stage left. Each are thanked for coming by Paul.

Mother: *So what do you reckon to that?*

Kath: *Good. I liked it.*

They leave the stage.

(Taken from Moore and Goodley, 1999)

UNDERSTANDING THE BAD REVIEW

Some of the factors which can give rise to a poor review
include:

- the trappings of professional territory
- dominance of a professional coterie
- imposition of personal preoccupations by professionals
- professional ineptitude
- imposition of a 'deficit' perspective (the client is positioned as the person with limitations)
- judgements of professionals taking precedence over the views of the person whom the review is ostensibly for
- lack of privacy
- lack of desirable options
- a professional rather than client-centred agenda

A GOOD REVIEW

(Description of a good review lasting 7 minutes 25 seconds)

The action proceeds more or less identically as in the bad review performance up until the point where the tea lady arrives. What happens next is strikingly different:

Client: *STOP! [Stands up, arm raised] ... I'LL SHOW YOU HOW I WANT MY REVIEW.*

Client tells the physio, *'I don't want you, you can go'.*

Physio shakes hands of staff and mum and leaves.

Client gets rid of tea lady, *'I'll have my tea later'.* Asks her mother to move her chair. Moves her and her chair by her own chair. Social and key worker, chairs in hands, are waved forward. The four chairs now form a square. She tells Paul, *'I'll sort you out later'.*

Audience laughs. ▶

Paul plays to the audience, *'Let me know when you are ready!'* Client does. She kicks him out, *'Can you leave please'.*

Then she turns to the onlookers and listeners. First, Alf and Tina.

Client: *And what are you doing? You can go!*

Then asks Paula and Peter: *And what are you doing? You can go!* [Audience laughs] [turns to face audience] *And this is how I want my review, in a nice little square, at home* [sits down].*Now can we get started? Thank you. Sooner we get it done the better.*

Mother: *Shall we find out first what suggestions the key worker and social worker have?*

Client: *Yeah.*

Mother: *Give us some things that Client might want to do please.*

Key worker: *There are different courses, sewing, computers …*

Social worker: *… caring for old people, child care.*

Mother: *Which of them would you like to do?* [addressing Client]

Client: *Old people – I don't like children they get on my nerves.*

[Mother and audience laugh]

Mother: *What, for five days of the week?*

Client: *No. Centre for two, go to the old people's home for three.*

Mother: *I suggest you get in touch with your key worker and set up a timetable. How does the key worker feel about this?*

Key worker: *Fine. I'll go along with it* [Smiles at the audience]

Mother: *Is there anything else?*

Client: *Eh ...*

Mother: *Is that it?*

Client: *Yeah.*

Mother: *Is there anything else you'd like to put forward?*

Client: *No... . And this is how I want it to be, I don't want it in any public place. I want it in my own home, where it is quiet and you get some peace.*

She walks off to *'There's no limit'.*

(Taken from Moore and Goodley, 1999)

UNDERSTANDING THE GOOD REVIEW

There are obvious qualitative differences between this and the last scene. It is informative to see performers preferring to be accompanied by an advocate, particularly in light of the many reviews that occur when professionals have actively fought for advocates not to attend (Booth 1991).

From this performance we learn that a good review:

- is directed by the client with the support of a trusted other
- is on the client's preferred territory
- sets aside professional allegiances
- is attentive and focused
- addresses professional incompetence
- is built on a 'capacity perspective' (the emphasis is on the strengths of the client and what they can do)
- is challenging of medical model dominance
- is private
- has discussion that includes all participants
- has paced dialogue and a number of options
- is client-centred rather than professional-centred

These performances confirm that practitioners have much to learn from people with learning difficulties about professional practices.

We are now just starting to find out the views of people with learning difficulties on their futures and how these are supported – mainly because they are becoming more articulate in public. The significance of knowing and valuing a person's own starting points cannot be stressed enough. Most people appreciate the opportunity to discuss their situation with someone whom they feel is genuinely concerned. Clearly, there is a need to be reliable and to establish open and comfortable processes of communication if anger, disappointment and disempowerment of older caregivers and people with learning difficulties is to be avoided.

PEOPLE WITH LEARNING DIFFICULTIES BRINGING ABOUT CHANGE

People with learning difficulties want a number of demands to be met. Decisions about the future are not simply a matter of choosing between, for example, long-term placement with another family, or occasional placement with another adult: there are many demands within these choices. Through our explorations of the views of people with learning difficulties we found that they want to be involved in deciding where they will live, who they will live with and so on.

An important factor for many people is that they should stay in the area they know and many want to stay in the house or flat they are used to. A sense of belonging and generally feeling accepted in any new environment is important, as is help in understanding the process of change: what is going to happen, when, with who involved, and so on. People are keen to make sure that contact with family members and friends can be maintained.

People with learning difficulties, like caregivers, stress that they want acceptance of their right to change their minds about future options, to be able to try a new living arrangement but move on again and try something different if needs be. Many people express a strong wish for parents to remain involved in their lives if they do leave home, which again echoes the preference of many caregivers.

Azra is in her 20s and lives with her parents. She likes going to a Day Centre from Monday to Friday to see friends and get out of the house, but gets very bored with the activities on offer. She also says that at the Day Centre people fight and she doesn't like that. Apart from going to the Day Centre she rarely gets out.

As her sister points out:

'[providers] need to organise some facilities where they can go at weekends, now that my parents are ageing, they can't take her out every weekend and that's what she likes to do, she want's to go out somewhere. She gets very upset and frustrated if she stays at home'.

Azra enjoys playing snooker and would like to be able to go and play in the evenings. She never spends any time away from her family. She does not receive any respite care and neither she or her family were aware respite care existed, though this is exactly what they would like.

Azra would like to have her own place. She would like to learn how to cook and do things which will help her to live independently. She has lived with her parents for a long time, and she is not getting out as much as she would like. Moving out would open up new possibilities. Her parents agree that the time is right for her to move:

'she wants to buy herself a house. We know that she can't look after herself, but we would like to have the facility where there is a person there ... and she can have the freedom'.

SELF-ADVOCACY

The growing worldwide self-advocacy movement has done much to create a vehicle for self-expression and direct control over their own affairs for people with learning difficulties. Self-advocacy involves a person expressing what they want as an individual. The self-advocacy movement in Britain is a living testament to the power of group activity by people with learning difficulties seeking to challenge institutionalised prejudice and oppressive jurisdiction in their lives (Goodley, 1998). Self-advocacy groups address numerous concerns expressed by people with learning difficulties, including housing, Day Centre Charges, rights to relationships and choice.

The conventional view of people with learning difficulties, which positions them as in need of 'special' attention and so different from others that they are almost totally excluded from mainstream life, is now being overturned by people with learning difficulties who are self-advocates. Self-advocates are increasingly informing policy-makers and bringing about long-overdue *social* change as they confirm that it is not people with learning difficulties who are the 'problem' for the rest of society but rather it is society itself which creates a problem for *them* in terms of their rightful inclusion in it (Moore and Goodley, 1999). The role of practitioners in the advancement of self-advocacy needs careful thought.

> *People see our disability only, they don't see our ability. We may have a handicap but we're not the handicap*
>
> **(Pat Worth, a Canadian self-advocate)**

Self-advocacy groups adopt a format not dissimilar to self-help groups. The main difference is that self-advocacy groups aspire to be user-led. This does not mean that a person without learning difficulties cannot attend a self-advocacy group and many self-advocacy groups do employ a person without learning difficulties as a facilitator. However, participants without learning difficulties have an obligation not to direct or overly influence the proceedings. They should not seek to set the agenda or shape the structure of the group, for example, to mirror a day-centre users-panel.

> *One day when Sue (the tutor) said we should do something, I said,* 'No, we don't have to do what you say'.   ➤

> *After a while it was decided that Sue should leave the*
> *group. Now we meet and we have a new adviser who is*
> *quiet and doesn't keep talking like Sue!*
> **(Atkinson and Williams, 1990, p. 190)**

It is also important that caregivers are encouraged to self-advocate. As we have seen they rarely feel they have a meaningful say and there is scope for practitioners to support caregivers in the development of personal advocacy. There are calls for increased cooperation between self-advocacy groups and practitioners and ways could be found of evolving forums where common issues can be taken up together. It is also important that people with learning difficulties and caregivers are enabled to participate in decision-making processes.

CITIZEN ADVOCACY

The Citizen Advocacy movement grew from questions being asked by caregivers in the United States in the 1960s about *'what will happen to my child when I'm gone?'* They decided that in the absence of family advocates, people with learning difficulties could be supported by a 'citizen advocate'.

> *Citizen advocates are unpaid, competent volunteers*
> *... independent of those providing direct service to*
> *people with disabilities [sic]. Working on a*
> *one-to-one basis they attempt to foster respect for the*
> *rights and dignity of those whose interests they*
> *represent. This may involve helping to express the*
> *individual's concerns and aspirations, obtaining*
> *day-to-day social, recreational, health and related*
> *services, and providing other practical and emotional*
> *support.*
> **(Citizen Advocacy Information & Training, 1996)**

The first citizen advocacy scheme was set up in the UK in 1981 by the Advocacy Alliance. Relationships are intended to be long-term but some citizen advocates are involved in crisis or short-term situations.

As well as being independent of services, citizen advocates are also independent of family and friends which is helpful if either party wishes to discuss things which may disturb relations either with the usual mediator or within relevant social groups. A useful example is where there may be conflict for the disabled person between their acceptance of the support they receive and the supporter who provides it;

> *'Pat doesn't like his key worker.'*
>
> **(Morris, 1993)**

The role of the citizen advocate is not an easy one, not least because the expectations of others are often ill-defined. Issues involving power, control and disablement at individual, group and societal levels are important and perhaps need airing more often. A service provider pointed out the importance of recognising power imbalance – a matter which we agree is crucial:

> *Power issues must be considered. The individuals in this case have never been asked before about their opinions on such areas and due to unequal balance of power between the two parties, may not be forthcoming and so become disempowered.*

- How can the seemingly counter needs of 'direct access', 'mediated encounters', 'full communication' and 'self-determination' be met?
- What responsibilities prevail upon practitioners wanting to redress the power balance in their interactions with people with learning difficulties and caregivers?
- How is it possible to begin breaking down barriers which threaten to restrict full involvement of all parties in your own work context?

There are 3 practice pointers for practitioners:

- citizen advocates and their representative agencies will provide allies for people with learning difficulties with whom you work – there are currently at least two hundred groups across the UK;
- setting up citizen advocacy schemes for caregivers could enable greater control over their own affairs for those who want somebody independent to work with them to secure services or uphold their rights;
- seeking out and supporting *self*-advocacy will create a culture for achieving excellence.

Taking action

**At the moment, we know more about what
researchers and practitioners think about policy and
practice for people with learning difficulties and older
caregivers than we know about what they think
themselves. This is a situation in need of redress and
further explorations need to become a constant
feature of practitioner activity:**

- what recommendations do current caregivers and people with learning difficulties you work with have for practitioners – both locally and nationally? How can you find out? Can support be gleaned for these aspirations from other disabled people and their representative organisations?
- how could these views be presented in order to stimulate change and to whom?
- who can be pressed to evolve new regular forums for accessing the views of people with learning difficulties and caregivers?
- what specific change(s) would make an immediate difference to people with learning difficulties and caregivers you work with?

RECOMMENDATIONS

The Uncertain Futures project brought together by Carol
Walker and Alan Walker to look at the situation of people
with learning difficulties and their ageing family caregivers
makes several recommendations for developing proactive
services which prevents crises, and we have built on these
here:

- develop a **database** of all family caregivers and a database of all people with learning difficulties receiving support – use this database to facilitate sharing knowledge, expertise and experience between practioners
- develop a comprehensive and regularly updated **information resource** for caregivers covering issues such as emergency ❧

- ◀ and respite procedures – which should also be made available in accessible formats for people with learning difficulties and for those with sensory impairments
- organise a **showcase of the range of future living options** – this could be through written materials, a photo montage, video, or event-based for example; working with the media can help spread information about new developments
- **enhance continuity** with a key worker of the service user's own choosing – formalise contingency plans and specify fail-safe arrangements so that problems do not escalate
- carry out **regular reviews** of the situation of caregivers and people with learning difficulties living together – which enable people to speak for themselves and which are characterised by careful listening and respect
- **agree plans for future care** – this helps counter the view that 'nothing is being done'; even if there are no guarantees, at least there will be indicators of what is wanted
- have **clear signposts indicating who is accountable** for what and encourage participation in monitoring and evaluation procedures
- ensure **appropriate training** for practitioners in facilitating self-determination for service users
- establish trust through earning it – **'rebuilding the confidence of people with learning difficulties and older caregivers in the paid service sector'.**

(Adapted from Walker and Walker, 1998)

COALITIONS

There is an increasing trend for establishing 'coalitions' of service users, practitioners and managers in order to create coordinated community care responses. Caregivers and people with learning difficulties with whom we have contact feel that such coalitions would improve standards by increasing the likelihood of their voices being heard and creating greater accountability. They believe a forum is required where they can articulate their concerns without these being compartmentalised into separate sets of concerns for people with learning difficulties, for caregivers and/or for older people. They feel that separating out the interests of people with learning difficulties and caregivers leads their situations to be viewed in relation to different priorities and parameters which means, in turn, that understanding of the interests of the whole family is fragmented or even lost. Following our research, caregivers, people with learning difficulties and practitioners – including purchasing managers – began to identify some of their goals for a local coalition.

> - To create a coordinated response to meet the self-determined needs of caregivers and people with learning difficulties
> - To develop service strategy which links organisations, individuals and their respective expertise together, within an agreed framework, underpinned by commitment to maximising the rights of caregivers and people with learning difficulties
> - To prioritise accountability to caregivers and people with learning difficulties
> - To provide a forum which encourages collaboration and debate between all key stakeholders and which is committed to producing practical outcomes from theoretical aspirations
> - To create a catalyst for best practice which currently exists, and for the implementation of sustainable change that will maximise best practice in the field
>
> **(Steering Group, Skelton et al, 1997)**

Such a list requires constant scrutiny and revision from time to time, but it has helped to focus attention on the importance of service users' *own starting* points in the planning, developing and running of local services. A coalition or similar structure offers participants the scope to build a continually evolving model of best practice which is expectant of, and responsive to change. This is important in the context of much uncertainty in the lives of older caregivers and people with learning difficulties. Caregivers and people with learning difficulties need collective strength. It is vital that they are fully and democratically involved in saying what their demands are and what solutions they endorse. They do not want decisions taken in their name. They want to play a full and proper role in creating them.

A set of questions which were originally posed to those interested in the links between disability politics and community care (Priestly, 1999) have been drawn on to further the thinking of practitioners here. They need to be interpreted in full view of the real pressures on practitioners and the necessity of finding empowering ways of working in the context of undeniable constraints – which is not going to be easy:

- In what ways does the community care agenda sustain disabling boundaries around caregivers and people with learning difficulties?
- How can caregivers and people with learning difficulties be supported in beginning to create change?
- How can caregivers and people with learning difficulties establish their expectations of practitioners and services?
- What is the best way to improve the quality of services to caregivers and people with learning difficulties? What outcomes will be most valued by service users?
- What barriers have to be removed to implement an agenda set by caregivers and people with learning difficulties with whom you work?

(Adapted from Priestly, 1999)

What would you want for yourself?
Whenever you are in doubt recall the face of the most struggling person with learning difficulties living with a family caregiver you have seen and ask yourself if the step you contemplate is going to make any difference to them ... will they gain anything by it?
Will it bring them greater control over their own life and destiny?
Do these questions alter your doubts?
Adaptation of words spoken by
Mahatma (M K) Gandhi

Appendix I
Legislation and entitlements

WHO ARE OLDER CAREGIVERS

**The Carers National Association, does not specify
what someone has to do to be defined as a caregiver,
stating only that**

> *'a carer is someone who provides a substantial
> amount of care on a regular basis.'*
> **(Carers National Association, 1996)**

The business of what constitutes 'a substantial amount' or
'a regular basis' is left for individuals to define. There is a
problem with this because people perceive and weigh up
their input in different ways. Lack of a tangible definition
places responsibility for knowing one's status as a
caregiver with those who are doing the caregiving but, as
stated in a newsletter for caregivers, most are

> *'too busy caring to have the luxury to think.'*
> **(Devine, 1999)**

These are thorny issues because, on the other hand, it
might be better that people should identify themselves in
order that the power of determining caregiver status is not
moved from individuals to providers. A real challenge for
practitioners lies in working through the ambivalent status
of many older caregivers in order to make sure that they
get the support for which they qualify.

STATUS AND ENTITLEMENTS

Being formally recognised as a caregiver is vital because it
helps to determine entitlements. At the time of writing, for
example, once it is established that a person provides

more than thirty-five hours of care a week, they may be eligible to receive benefit entitlements and financial discounts such as Invalid Care Allowance (ICA) and the Carers Council Tax Discount.

However as the information box shows, eligibility for older caregivers is neither straight-forward nor unproblematic:

Invalid Care Allowance

ICA is only available to caregivers if:

- they are between sixteen and under sixty-five
- they are looking after a person for at least thirty-five hours a week
- the person they are looking after is getting Attendance Allowance or Disability Living Allowance at the middle or higher rate for help with personal care
- the caregiver earns less than fifty pounds net a week

Notes:

For each week that the person is paid ICA they will get a National Insurance (NI) credit (Class 1). This may help the person to qualify for other social security benefits in the future including retirement pension.

It is important to note that caregivers who are over sixty-five, or those who are caring for people who do not claim middle to higher rates of AA and DLA Care, are not recognised as caregivers by the state. These people are missing out on benefits and NI stamps, despite care commitments which may mean they are not able to work.

The 1999 National Carers Strategy aims to give caregivers increased support and recognition partly through the proposed introduction of a second pension. This recognises that care commitments preclude many older caregivers from accruing enough National Insurance contributions for an adequate income in later life. While this is a welcome initiative – and much talked about at the time of writing – practitioners need to be aware that it may or may not actually happen since there are no plans to have it in place before the year 2050.

Many people who provide care for adult relatives find themselves having to push back the boundaries of coping in order to avoid their family becoming financially worse off. It is possible for older caregivers and people with learning difficulties to develop and purchase their own care package:

Direct Payments for people with learning difficulties

The aim of Direct Payments is to help people live independently. Instead of automatically receiving services through Social Services, disabled people can be given money direct (a 'Direct Payment') to organise their own support. This gives greater choice and control over services. The money received can be used by the person to either pay an agency to provide the necessary support, or to employ their own staff. To qualify for a Direct Payment, the person must be over eighteen and under sixty-five and must receive, or have been assessed as being eligible to receive, 5 or more hours of community care services.

Independent Living Fund (ILF 93)

ILF 93 is a trust set up and financed by central government. Like Direct Payments, the money awarded from ILF93 must be used to employ one or more people for personal or domestic support. There are a number of criteria which the person claiming has to meet, including being over sixteen and under sixty-six, receiving the higher rate of Disability Living Allowance care Component, and receiving at least two hundred pounds worth of services a week from their Local Authority.

Direct Payments for caregivers

As part of the National Carers Strategy (1999), the possibility of caregivers receiving Direct Payments or a similar credit scheme themselves is being explored. This will help to ensure that caregivers receive the support they want and need rather than just what is commonly available. However, at the time of writing it is not known whether this will be limited to those under sixty-five which will therefore exclude older caregivers.

Also, and perhaps more inauspicious, Direct payments for caregivers will require legislation to be changed and there has been no indication of this being prioritised.

Entitlements can and do vary, sometimes dramatically, from one caregiver to the next. Consulting with the local welfare rights officer will help uncover any entitlements possibly not being claimed and to examine potential entitlement pitfalls facing individual claimants in the future. Many local authorities employ benefits advisors. Useful booklets detailing other sources of advice are published by the British Institute of Learning Disabilities (listed below). Organisation such as MENCAP, Carers National and Carers Centre advise older caregivers and their representatives.

Practice pointers include:

- find out where to go for advice
- the Disability Rights Handbook gives clear guidelines and can keep practitioners up to date
- think about who else can help – advising practitioners, advising caregivers and advising people with learning difficulties

INVALUABLE SOURCES OF INFORMATION

Disability Rights Handbook Available from local libraries or can be purchased from Disability Alliance ERA. Tel: 0171 247 8765

British Institute of Learning Disabilities (1998) *Working with Older Carers: Guidance for Service Providers in Learning Disability* BILD Publications. Available from BILD

British Institute of Learning Disabilities Leaflet *Who Can Help Me Now? Advice and Information for Older Carers* Available from BILD

Walker, C and Walker, A (1998) *Uncertain Futures: People with learning difficulties and their ageing family carers* East Sussex, Pavilion Publishing / Joseph Rowntree Foundation

Appendix II
Useful Contacts

**Many of these contacts are national centres which will
be able to put readers in touch with local agencies**

SUPPORT FOR CARE GIVERS FIRST

Carers Line
  Tel: 0345 573 3691
Carers National Association
  20–25 Glasshouse Yard, London EC1 4JS
  Tel: 0171 490 8818
Sharing Caring Project
  Norfolk Lodge, Park Grange Road, Sheffield S2 3QF
  Tel: 0114 275 8879
Age Concern
  Astral House, 1268 London Road, London SW16 4ER
  Tel: 0181 679 8000
Help the Aged
  St James Walk, Clerkenwell Green, London EC1R OBE
  Tel: 0171 253 0454
Princess Royal Trust for Carers
  142 Minories, London E3N 1LB
Crossroads Care Attendant Scheme
  10, Regent Place, Rugby, Warwickshire CV21 2PN

SUPPORT FOR PEOPLE WITH LEARNING DIFFICULTIES FIRST

Citizen Advocacy Information and Training
  164 Lee Valley Techno Park, Ashley Road, Tottenham Hall,
  London N17 9LN
  Tel: 0181 880 5445
People First
  Instrument House, 207–215 Kings Cross Road, London WC1X 9DB
  Tel: 0171 713 6400
National Centre for Independent Living
  250 Kennington Lane, London SE11 5RD
  Tel: 0171 587 1663
Values Into Action
  Oxford House, Derbyshire Street, London E2 6HG
  Tel: 0171 729 5436

SUPPORT FOR PEOPLE WITH LEARNING DIFFICULTIES AND THEIR OLDER CARE-GIVERS

Enable
6th Floor, 7 Buchanan Street, Glasgow G1 3HL
Tel: 0141 226 4541

MENCAP
123 Golden Lane, London EC1Y 0RT
Tel: 0171 454 0454

MENCAP in Wales
31, Lambourne Crescent, Cardiff Business Park, Llanishen, Cardiff CF4 5GG
Tel: 01222 747588

MENCAP in Northern Ireland
Segal House, 4, Annadale Avenue, Belfast BT7 3JH
Tel: 01232 691351

Contact A Family
170 Tottenham Court Road, London W1P 0HA
Tel: 0171 383 3555

British Institute of Learning Disability
Wolverhampton Road, Kidderminster, Worcestershire DY10 3PP
Tel: 01562 850251

OTHER SOURCES OF SUPPORT

Direct Payments – Contact Your Local Social Services Department
For information on receiving Direct Payments, write to:
Department of Health, PO Box 410, Wetherby LS23 7LN

Independent Living Fund
PO Box 183, Nottingham NG8 3RD
Tel: 0115 942 8191

Federation Of Local Supported Living Groups
5 The Bowlings, Springfield, Wigan WN6 7B4
Tel: 01942 235 135

The Disability Law Service
Room 214, 2nd Floor, 49–51 Bedford Row, London WC1R 4LR
Tel: 0171 831 8031

Association of Lawyers for People with Learning Difficulty
115–123 Golden Lane, London EC1Y 0RT
Tel: 0171 454 0454

References

Alldred, P. (1996) Whose expertize? Conceptualizing resistance to advice about childrearing. In Burman, E, Aitken, G, Alldred, P, Allwood, R, Billington, T, Goldberg, B, Gordo Lopez, A J, Heenan, C, Marks, D and Warner, S *Psychology, Discourse Practice* London, Taylor and Francis

Aspis, S (1997) 'I'll Have a Banana' *Community Living* 1 October, pp14–15

Atkinson, D and Williams,F (eds.) (1990) *'Know me as I am' An Anthology of Prose, Poetry and Art by People with Learning Difficulties* Kent, Hodder and Stoughton in association with the Open University and MENCAP

Bashford, L, Townsley, R, and Williams, C. (1995) 'Parallel Text: Making Research Accessible to People with Intellectual Disabilities' *International Journal of Disability, Development and Education* 42(3), pp211–20

Barnes, C (1990) *Cabbage Syndrome: The Social Construction of Dependence* London, The Falmer Press

Beazley, S, Moore, M and Benzie, D (1997) 'Involving Disabled People in Research' in Barnes, C and Mercer, G *Doing Disability Research* Leeds, Disability Press

Beazley, S (2000) Accessing perspectives of children who do not use the majority language. In Moore, M. (Ed) *Insider Perspectives on Inclusion: raising voices, raising issues* Sheffield, Philip Armstrong Publications

BILD (British Institute of Learning Disabilities) (1998) *Working with Older Carers: Guidance for Service Providers in Learning Disability* Worcestershire, BILD Publications

Blair, T (1999) *Caring About Carers: A National Strategy for Carers Policy Briefing* London, Carers National Association

Booth, W (1991) 'A Cry for Help in the Wilderness' *The Health Service Journal* 14 February pp26–27

Booth, T and Booth, W (1994) *Parenting Under Pressure: Mothers and Fathers with Learning Difficulties* Buckingham, Open University Press

Carers National Association (1996) *New Rights for Carers. The Carers Recognition and Services Act – What it means for carers* London, Carers National Association

Carers National Association (1997) *Still Battling? The Carers Act One Year On* London, Carers National Association

Citizen Advocacy Information and Training (1996) *Citizen Advocacy Information Pack* London, Citizen Advocacy Information and Training

Devine, S (1999) '"Caring About Cares": A summary and reaction from Manchester Carer Centre Manager' *Manchester Carers Newsletter Issue 20*

Goodley, D (1997) 'Locating Self-advocacy in Models of Disability: Understanding Disability in the Support of Self-advocates with Learning Difficulties' *Disability and Society* 12(3) pp367–380

Goodley, D (1998) 'Supporting People with Learning Difficulties in Self-advocacy Groups and Models of Disability' *Health and Social Care in the Community* 6(5) pp438-446

Goodley, D (2000) 'Accessing the Views of People with Learning Difficulties' in Moore, M (Ed) *Insider Perspectives on Inclusion: raising voices, raising issues* Sheffield, Philip Armstrong Publications

Kagan, C and Lewis, S (1996) 'Families with Parents who have Multiple Commitment' in Moore, M, Sixsmith, J and Knowles, K (eds) *Children's Reflections on Family Life* Lewis, Falmer Press

Lewis, S, Kagan, C, Heaton, P and Cranshaw, M (1999) 'Economic and Psychological Benefits from Employment: the experiences and perspectives of mothers of disabled children' *Disability and Society* 14 (4) pp561-575

McDonald, A (1999) *Challenging Local Authority Decisions* Birmingham, Venture Press

Moore, M and Goodley, D (1999) *People with Learning Difficulties and Performing Arts: maximising the benefits of participation* University of Sheffield, Inclusive Education Research Centre Occasional Report

Moore, M, Beazley, S and Maelzer, J (1998) *Researching Disability Issues* Buckingham, The Open University Press

Morris, J (1993) *Independent Lives? Community care and disabled people* Basingstoke, Hants, Macmillan

Morris, J (1997) *Community Care: Working in partnership with service users* Birmingham, Venture Press

Oliver, M (1996) *Understanding Disability: From Theory to Practice* London: Macmillan

Oliver, M (1999) *Social Inclusion and Disabled People: Implications for Education?* Public Lecture at University of Sheffield, Ranmoor Hall

Priestly M (1999) *Disability Politics and Community Care* London, Jessica Kingsley

Read, J (2000) *Disability, the Family and Society. Listening to mother* Buckingham. The Open University Press

Rodgers, J (1999) 'Trying to Get it Right: undertaking research involving people with learning difficulties' *Disability and Society* 14(4) pp421-433

Skelton, J, Moore, M (1999) 'The Role of Self Advocacy in Work for People with Learning Difficulties' *Community, Work and Family* 2(2) pp133-145

Skelton, J and Moore, M, Beazley, S, Patient, M, and Maelzer, J (1997) *Listening to Older Care-Givers: Research into Aspirations for Support* IOD 8/97, Manchester Metropolitan University

Sutcliffe, J and Simons, K (1993) *Self-advocacy and Adults with Learning Difficulties: Contexts and Debates* Leicester, The National Institute of Adult Continuing Education in Association with The Open University Press

Swain, J, Gillman, M and French, S (1999) *Confronting Disabling Barriers: towards making organisations accessible* Birmingham, Venture Press

Walker, C and Walker, A (1998) *Uncertain Futures: People with learning difficulties and their ageing family carers* East Sussex, Pavilion Publishing / Joseph Rowntree Foundation

OTHER TITLES AVAILABLE IN THIS SERIES

Challenging Local Authority Decisions *Ann McDonald*

This book examines how dissatisfaction with outcomes can be used positively to challenge local authority decisions. Sometimes it will be the service provision that is challenged; at other times, it will be the way in which that decision is reached and the procedures used which are considered oppressive or unfair. All practitioners should know how to challenge local authority decisions through use of complaints procedures; default powers; referrals to the Ombudsman; or through the courts. In doing so good practice is reinforced, legality is tested and rights upheld.

ISBN: 1 86178 015 X

Child Protection and Domestic Violence
Audrey Mullender & Thangam Debbonaire

A child-centred and women-centred approach to examining the impact of domestic violence on children, together with ways in which professionals can most helpfully respond. The book summmarises what is known about domestic violence and its effects on children, and outlines key approaches in UK and overseas practice to intervening to protect, support and work directly with children whose mothers are being abused. The book is a 'must read' for social workers, community nurses, teachers youth weorkers and everyone who works with children and/or families.

ISBN: 1 86178 042 7

Community Care: working in partnership with service users *Jenny Morris*

This book sets out four principles for working in partnership with people who need support in their daily lives: entitlement; the social model for disability; needs-led assessment; and promoting choice and control. Drawing on the wealth of research and information now available about how to work in ways which empower people. Examples are given relating to all the community care service user groups – older people, people with learning difficulties, those with physical/sensory impairment and people who use mental health services.

ISBN: 1 873878 91 5

Confronting Disabling Barriers: towards making organisations accessible
John Swain, Maureen Gillman & Sally French

Little has been written for social workers and other professionals on disabling barriers within institutions. This guide draws upon the discipline of disability studies to assist practitioners who seek to make their organisations accessible to disabled people. This guide analyses institutional discrimination against disabled people and highlights ways in which organisations can become more accessible to them. The authors use a civil rights perspective underpinned by the social model of disability.

ISBN: 1 86178 027 3

Deafness and the Hearing *Jennifer Harris*

This book invites a radical change in the majority view on Deafness. The author spent four years studying an organisation of Deaf people in the UK and analysing the reactions of the Hearing majority. The results were dramatic; descriptions of stigmatism, oppressive practice and prejudicial attitudes emerged. The message of the book is that it is not deafness itself which determines social exclusion but entrenched prejudicial attitudes of 'the Hearing'.

ISBN: 1 86178 016 8

Dealing with Aggression   *Brian Littlechild*

How can aggression and violence to staff in social work and social care settings be managed? This book sets out in a clear and concise manner an integrated approach to the wide range of problems presented by aggression and violence. It covers risk assessment and coping strategies from the perspectives of the different individuals involved, and of staff groups and agencies. The best strategies for dealing with aggression face to face are presented, as are ways we can most effectively reduce risk. For students and experienced workers alike, this book gives a comprehensive account of how to increase safety at work.

ISBN: 1 873878 98 2

Dilemmas of Financial Assessment   *Greta Bradley & Jill Manthorpe*

The implementation of the NHS and Community Care Act 1990 has impacted on the lives of service users and social workers. This book explores one important area of change: the increasing emphasis on assessing users' financial circumstances in order to maximise their incomes but also to establish their ability to pay for services. For many social workers this is new ground. Some experienced social workers feel anxious and torn between the new culture of community care and the values they associate with traditional social work tasks.

ISBN: 1 873878 90 7

Down's Syndrome and Dementia   *Diana Kerr*

This book defines good practice in needs assessment and the provision of services for the growing number of people with Down's Syndrome and Dementia. It is based on a social model which demands that we see the person first and the disease second. It gives many practical examples of ways in which workers and carers can intervene to support people and avoid behaviour and practices which disempower and can harm. It will be relevant to social workers, social care workers, community nurses, carers, staff in supported accommodation and anyone working in community settings.

ISBN: 1 86178 017 6

Drugs, Children and Families   *Jane Mounteney & Harry Shapiro*

This book aims to demystify the drug phenomenon, and increase social workers' knowledge of drug use, by providing a range of up-to-date information about drugs and their effects, by exploring ways drug use may arise as an issue for clients and social services departments and through exploration of a range of social work interventions. *Drugs, Children and Families* draws on relevant research where this exists and highlights a number of concerns, particularly in relation to interventions and provision for young people with drug use problems.

ISBN: 1 86178 013 3

Family Support   *Ruth Gardner*

Family support has attracted much less attention in terms of research and development than the more clearly defined systems for children in need of statutory protection and/or those looked after by local authorities. Yet it is a legal requirement of the Children Act (England and Wales) 1989, backed up by the UN Convention on the Rights of the Child. This book describes the essential elements of good family support and gives examples of research, planning, budget management and evaluated practice. It is essential reading for managers and practitioners, commissioning or providing these services, in all settings.

ISBN: 1 86178 026 5